A Reference Guide to Surviving Nature

GEAR • WILDLIFE • WEATHER • FIRST AID
OUTDOOR PREPARATION AND REMEDIES

DR. NICOLE APELIAN

&

SHAWN CLAY

"Keep close to Nature's heart... and break clear away, once in awhile, and climb a mountain or spend a week in the woods. Wash your spirit clean."

– John Muir

DISCLAIMER

This guide is intended to be a general resource for the prevention and treatment of the various possible plant / insect / animal / weather encounters while outdoors. It is not intended to be all-inclusive, rather dealing mainly with the plants, insects, and animals most commonly found throughout the continental United States. There may be various species or varieties present in your specific area that are not covered that you should still be aware of. I would encourage the reader to research the various threats that may be present in their region. Resources to do this are available in the appendix section of the guide.

This guide is not intended to be taken as official medical advice. Please consult your physician for any official diagnosis or treatment that may be necessary. If you are interested in becoming certified in first aid or other forms of life-saving treatment, contact your local Red Cross or other emergency management group for certification classes in your area.

ABOUT THE AUTHORS

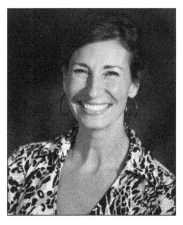

DR. NICOLE APELIAN is a wilderness living skills and prepping/emergency preparedness instructor. She is also an herbalist and has a deep knowledge of medicinal plants. At home in the Pacific Northwest, she makes her own herbal medicines from local plants as part of her healthy living strategy. Nicole thrives as a personal wellness and life coach helping people develop personalized holistic life plans, especially as related to autoimmune issues, and has her own herbal medicinal apothecary line. Nicole was a challenger on the second and fifth seasons of the History Channel's TV series "Alone", where she thrived in the wilderness totally solo with little more than her knife and her wits. She teaches workshops on her land in the Pacific NW, and also travels to teach skills across the globe. For more about Nicole, please visit www.nicoleapelian.com.

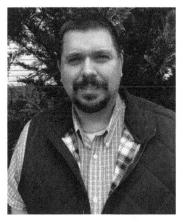

SHAWN CLAY is an outdoor writer, focusing mainly on preparedness and self-reliance. He is a member of the Walker County, Georgia C.E.R.T. and seeks to spread the message about the importance of preparation in both the home and the community. An avid hunter and fisherman, he prefers any activity that keeps him and his family in the great outdoors. He resides in Flintstone, Georgia in the foothills of beautiful Lookout Mountain with his wife and two children. He is available to speak to groups about the importance of preparation and how to get started. To contact Shawn, send a friend request on Facebook or email him directly at: smokey30725@gmail.com.

TABLE OF CONTENTS

DISCLAIMER

ABOUT THE AUTHORS

CHAPTER 1: BASIC CONSIDERATIONS 1
- COMMUNICATION / SIGNALING 2
- FIRST AID 2
- KNIFE / MULTITOOL... 3
- FLASHLIGHT 3
- FIRE-STARTING 4
- SHELTER 4
- WATER 5
- FOOD.. 5

CHAPTER 2: POISONOUS PLANTS 7
- POISON IVY 7
- POISON OAK.. 8
- POISON SUMAC.. 9
- STINGING NETTLE 10
- WOOD NETTLE 11
- RAGWEED 11
- GIANT HOGWEED.. 12
- WILD PARSNIP 13

CHAPTER 3: INFURIATING INSECTS 16
ANTS.. 16
- ACROBAT ANTS 17
- CARPENTER ANTS 18
- PAVEMENT ANTS 18
- FIRE ANTS 18
BEES 19
- HONEY BEE 19
- AFRICAN BEE 20
- BUMBLE BEE 20
WASPS 22
- BALD-FACED HORNET.. 23
- EUROPEAN HORNET 23
- PAPER WASPS 25
- YELLOWJACKETS.. 25
MOSQUITOS 26
CATERPILLARS 27
- SADDLEBACK CATERPILLAR 27
- HAG MOTH CATERPILLAR 28
- PUSS CATERPILLAR... 28
- STINGING ROSE CATERPILLAR 28
- SPINY ELM CATERPILLAR.. 29
- WHITE FLANNEL CATERPILLAR....................................... 29

• CROWNED SLUG CATERPILLAR 29
• IO MOTH CATERPILLAR 30
• WHITE MARKED TUSSOCK MOTH CATERPILLAR 30
• BUCK MOTH CATERPILLAR 30
SCORPIONS 31
SPIDERS 32
• RECLUSES 33
• WIDOWS 34
• HOBO SPIDER 35
• YELLOW SAC SPIDER 35
BITING FLIES 36
• DEER FLY 36
• HORSE FLY 37
• STABLE FLY 37
• BLACK FLY 38
• GREENHEAD FLY 38
• BITING MIDGE 38
TICKS 39
• AMERICAN DOG TICK 40
• BLACKLEGGED TICK 40
• BROWN DOG TICK 41
• GULF COAST TICK 42
• LONE STAR TICK 42
• ROCKY MOUNTAIN WOOD TICK 43
• WESTERN BLACKLEGGED TICK 43
CENTIPEDES 44
LEECHES 45
CHIGGERS 46

CHAPTER 4: CRITTERS THAT WALK, STALK AND SLITHER 48
• MOUNTAIN LIONS 49
• BROWN/GRIZZLY BEARS 50
• BLACK BEARS 53
• WOLVES 55
• WILD BOAR 57
• RACOONS 60
• SKUNKS 61
• BATS 62
• COYOTES 63
• FOXES 64
• RATTLESNAKES 66
• DIAMONDBACK RATTLESNAKE 67
• TIMBER / CANEBRAKE RATTLESNAKE 67
• PYGMY RATTLESNAKE 68
• PRAIRIE RATTLESNAKE 69
• SIDEWINDER RATTLESNAKE 70
• COPPERHEAD 72
• COTTONMOUTH 73

• CORAL SNAKE 76

• ALLIGATORS 78

CHAPTER 5: WICKED WEATHER 81

• FROSTBITE 81

• HYPOTHERMIA 83

• CRAMPS 84

• HEAT EXHAUSTION 85

• HEAT STROKE 85

• SUNBURN 86

• DEHYDRATION 87

• HAZARDS 88

• WILDFIRES 89

• LIGHTNING 90

CHAPTER 6: THE BASICS OF WILDERNESS FIRST AID 92

CHAPTER 7: PLANNING YOUR NEXT OUTDOOR ADVENTURE 96

CHAPTER 8: IN CLOSING 99

APPENDIX / RESOURCE GUIDE 101

• KNIVES / MULTITOOLS 101

• BASIC EMERGENCY FIELD KIT & CHECKLIST 103

• FLARES 104

• SMOKE GRENADES 104

• EMERGENCY LOCATOR BEACONS 105

• FLASHLIGHTS 105

• SIX COMMON MEDICINAL PLANTS & LICHENS 106

• MULLEIN 106

• PLANTAIN 106

• STINGING NETTLE 107

• USNEA 107

• WILLOW 108

• YARROW 108

• DR. NICOLE'S NATURAL RECIPES FOR PAIN RELIEF 109

• NATURAL BUG & TICK REPELLANT SPRAY 110

• GEAR SELECTION 111

• FIRST AID TRAINING 112

• RECOMMENDED READING 114

• CHILDREN & THE OUTDOORS 116

• MAPS 117

• LOCAL PRIVATE RESOURCES & EDUCATION 117

• SPECIAL THANKS 119

• PHOTOGRAPH AND COVER DESIGN CREDITS 119

• NOTES 124

• POCKET VERSION OF BASIC EMERGENCY FIELD KIT & CHECKLIST .. 135

CHAPTER ONE

CAREFUL CONSIDERATIONS

When planning a vacation, very few of us would simply jump in the car and start driving. Most of us put some degree of forethought and planning into any type of trip that we undertake. The same principle should, to a degree, apply to any trip into the great outdoors. While that's not to say that a week's worth of planning should go into a spontaneous afternoon hike or dip in the creek, there is a certain amount of due diligence that needs to be done before striking off on an adventure. Those of us with children know this concept well. This chapter will address some of the basic considerations that should be reviewed and addressed before striking off into the great unknown. As the old saying goes, an ounce of prevention is worth a pound of cure.

Most outdoorsmen and women have some form of basic essentials on them at all times, be it in a backpack, belt pouch, or simply in their pockets. While it is sometimes easy to go overboard and inadvertently pack enough gear that you look like your are embarking on a modern-day Lewis and Clark expedition, the concept of minimalism can certainly be of great help. Often times, a small day pack is all that is needed to carry the necessary preventative gear. Your contents may vary depending on your particular set of circumstances, but here is a summation of what should be included in your gear (adapted from Nicole Apelian's Basic Emergency Field Kit. A complete checklist is included in the appendix).

COMMUNICATION & SIGNALING

Most, if not all of us, likely have a cell phone within arm's reach of us at all times. While the purpose of getting out into nature is often to escape the constant buzzing of incoming texts and emails, it is a good idea to take your cell phone with you, even if you power it down. In the event that you become lost or injured with your cell phone you can call for help, determine your physical location via GPS, and have illumination in the event you have to travel at night. A charging method such as a battery bank or small solar charger is a wonderful addition as well.

If you choose not to take your cell phone, a quality whistle is something that can be effectively used to signal for help should you become stranded or injured. In addition, letting someone know where you are going and how long you plan to be out is essential, as is signing in at a trailhead if you are in a park. This way, your loved ones, friends and park rangers have a frame of reference if you don't arrive back on time and that information can be crucial to search and rescue teams if the need for them to deploy arises.

A neon signaling flag or the like is also key. Search and rescue has great difficulty finding people who blend in to their environment so having a neon orange flag or piece of clothing may save your life. Also, having local area maps is always a good idea, as is a map compass, since the reflective lens can also be used as a signaling device. Additionally, a small signal mirror can serve as an aid when trying to catch the attention of rescue personnel. Having multiple ways of being seen will definitely increase your odds of being spotted or heard by rescue teams.

FIRST AID

This is often the most overlooked gear that should be present. And please don't simply buy the 99-cent travel-size first aid kit that contains two bandaids and an alcohol wipe. Should you, or someone in your group, actually need to use it, you will find that you are woefully unprepared. We will get into the particulars of what should go into your kit in a later chapter, but suffice to say, this is one area you do not want to skimp on.

At a minimum, one should include the following:

- Emergency Medication: anti-diarrheal, aspirin, ibuprofen, Benadryl or similar antihistamine, any prescription medication you need on a daily basis.

- Bandages: a small assortment of large and small bandaids and butterfly closures, along with a pair of tweezers. A compression bandage (such as an Israeli bandage) and Chito-Sam bandage are recommended as well. These are both excellent for stopping blood flow for major, possibly lethal wounds. For arterial bleeds a tourniquet is needed (please get proper training for use).

- Tourniquet (the RevMedX and the SWAT-T are recommended)

- Small tube or tin of first aid salve

- Alcohol wipes - can be used to sterilize a wound, and also serve as a fire starter

KNIFE / MULTITOOL

If you are like us, you don't leave the house without at least a good pocket knife clipped to your pants or shorts. A knife is one of the most useful tools that you can have on you. Likewise, a multitool can come in very handy in a variety of situations. In the appendix section, you will find a breakdown of some of our recommended knives and tools that will fit any budget. If you spend enough time in the outdoors, you will come to learn that this little bit of weight is more than justified when you need it. A good blade can be worth its weight in gold. A lightweight fixed blade along with a smaller secondary knife / saw combo can come in quite handy. In addition, a small sewing kit gives one the ability to make field repairs to clothing, tents, etc.

FLASHLIGHT

Any outdoor gear should include a good quality flashlight along with a spare battery. With technology advancing, the size of flashlights continues to shrink as their lumen output continues to increase. As a result, the days of carrying a bulky spotlight or that 6 D Cell Maglite are over. Many companies now offer pint-sized lights that put out enough illumination to guide in a 747 jetliner. Some of our recommendations are found in the appendix section as well.

FIRE-STARTING

While none of us plan to get lost while outdoors, it happens to thousands of people every year. Having the ability to successfully start a fire can be a game-changer. Not only is it an effective way to maintain warmth and serve as a signal beacon, but a good fire has positive psychological benefits, as well as warding off potential predators. While some of us might want to channel our inner caveman and vigorously rub two sticks together in an attempt to start a roaring fire, the reality is that there are much more efficient methods of getting a fire going in an emergency. There are many products available, but the below items are recommended for anyone venturing into the wilderness:

- Ferro rod
- Lighter
- Fire-starting tinder
- Fresnel lens

For your emergency gear, remember that two is one, and one is none. Always carry more than one method of reliably lighting a fire with you at all times.

SHELTER

Being lost in the woods is no fun. Being lost in the woods and soaking wet is even less fun. Packing a poncho in your gear can also be useful just to keep you dry on that short day hike, and an emergency blanket can ensure that you retain heat and stay warm should you have to spend an unexpected night in the woods. Hypothermia can set in quickly, so it's recommended that one have the necessary means to prevent it. **Here are some suggestions:**

- Paracord (20' minimum)
- Wire saw to cut firewood, shelter poles, etc. A larger saw is good for your vehicle.
- Emergency poncho
- Emergency tarp / shelter sheet. A larger tarp can be kept in your vehicle.
- Mylar blanket (sometimes referred to as a space or emergency blanket)

WATER

Out of all gear considerations, this is probably the most important. Whether you plan to be out for an hour or all day, you definitely need to include a water source in order to stay hydrated. While a store brand bottle of water may suffice for a quick trip out, you may want to consider, once again, what would happen if your quick trip turned into an extended outing. Manufacturers such as Camelbak make daypacks with an integrated bladder that can carry multiple liters of water. In addition, many companies make reusable water bottles now that have an integrated cartridge for purifying water from questionable sources such as a creek or a river. We recommend one of these so that the option to refill as needed is available, without having to worry about a waterborne illness. A lot of waterborne illnesses result in cases of diarrhea, which can quickly lead to dehydration and become a life-threatening situation. At the very least, carry iodine tablets and drop some in to ensure that the bacteria and viruses are neutralized.

Of course, traditional water purifiers are an option, but many will not want the additional bulk or weight. That being said, Sawyer makes a very lightweight one (Sawyer mini), which is what we both carry with our everyday gear. We also include some small water storage bags, which allow you to keep more on hand should you have to make a temporary camp. Having water for drinking and water for cooking can make an emergency situation a lot more tolerable.

We recommend that you carry a single-sided stainless or titanium water bottle with your gear. This gives you the ability to boil water should the need arise. This is something that cannot be done in a plastic bottle or with an insulated steel water bottle. Many outdoor enthusiasts choose a water bottle kit that incorporates a nesting cup that can be used exclusively for cooking. While some of this sounds like a lot of gear to be packed, if done correctly, it can take up minimal room and weight. If needed, it will be well worth the forethought and additional bulk.

FOOD

On the subject of food, don't go overboard. In a situation where you are lost or stranded, food will actually take a back seat to water and shelter. A good compromise would be to take along some dried fruit and nuts, pemmican, or a granola bar or two. These lightweight options will keep you going when your stomach starts to rumble.

In addition, having a little bit of snare wire (24-28 gauge brass is recommended) along with a small fishing kit (hooks, line, sinkers) will allow you to hopefully procure food should your trip turn into a true survival situation.

These basic essentials should be present anytime one is venturing into the wilderness. The combined weight of these items can easily be kept below 10 pounds, therefore not interfering with your enjoyment of the journey. Of course, every reader's needs will be different, so you must determine what works best for your situation. You may want to include bug spray, sunblock, or any number of different items. Just ensure that you aren't adding so much that your pack becomes a hassle to take along. A bulky pack that winds up being left in the car will do you absolutely no good.

CHAPTER TWO

POISONOUS PLANTS

Nature is full of plants and flowers that can be beneficial and gorgeous to look at. The resources that they provide are countless. However, there are plants and vines that can be hazardous to us as well. This chapter will delve into the various types of hazardous plants that may be encountered in the wilderness. Our appendix also has a section on common medicinal plants that are known as curatives.

POISON IVY

Most of us are familiar with the old saying "leaves of three, let them be." Poison ivy is prevalent over much of the country and can be found in clusters on the ground and in vines that wrap around trees and other foliage. The distinctive three leaf pattern helps to identify it, but often we are exposed before we realize it. The plant contains a compound called urushiol, and it can be found in all parts of the plant, from the leaves, berries, and all the way down to the roots. When skin is exposed to urushiol, a red, blistering rash is the result. The duration of the rash depends on the amount of exposure. Some cases can be minor, while others spread to larger areas of the body and can be quite irritating. There are numerous home remedies and natural remedies that can be used to treat the symptoms and speed up the heal-

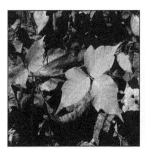 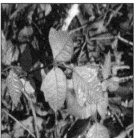 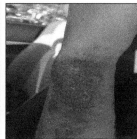

ing time. In addition, corticosteroid creams and sprays can help to reduce the inflammation and the incessant itching. In extreme cases, a doctor may prescribe a shot or prescription medication to bring the rash under control. A word of caution to anyone looking to clear property: the burning of poison ivy can cause the urushiol to become airborne. The inhalation of the smoke can cause internal irritation and can become serious very quickly. The photo on the right shows a victim of inhaled poison ivy during the burning of brush.

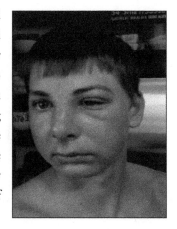

Fortunately, there are a number of options to avoid the discomfort that comes with exposure to poison ivy. There are several over the counter sprays and creams that can be applied to the skin before exposure to the plant that help prevent the urushiol from absorbing into the skin. I have a good friend who works for a utility company and they are issued bottles of Tecnu brand lotion and apply it to any exposed areas of skin before working in heavily wooded areas. Utility crews are constantly exposed to the plant, but have very good results with the preventive topical lotion. Other ways to avoid exposure are long sleeves and tucking pant legs into socks to ensure that there are few open areas to absorb the urushiol. If you have been in an area with lots of poison ivy, it's best to shower immediately to remove any residual urushiol and wash the clothes you were wearing.

Natural remedies include cool compresses with lavender oil, helichrysum oil, black tea, aloe vera, apple cider vinegar and/or witch hazel. Immediately washing the affected area with soap and water will help a lot as will oatmeal baths (grind up the oatmeal, put in a stocking or cheesecloth and put into your bath) and baking soda baths. Internal supplements such as stinging nettle, echinacea (unless you have an autoimmune disorder) and Vitamin C can also help.

POISON OAK

Like poison ivy, poison oak can be identified by its distinctive three leaf pattern. Various species are found from coast to coast. It has yellow flowers and the berries are somewhat fuzzy, where poison ivy berries are smooth. Like poison ivy, all parts

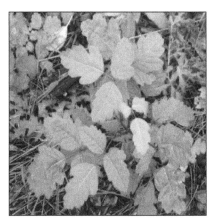 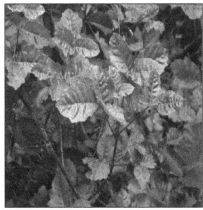

of poison oak contain urushiol. The rash and symptoms are essentially the same as poison ivy, as are the treatments. Care should be taken with clearing and burning brush containing poison oak, as inhalation can have the same dangerous results as inhaling poison ivy smoke.

POISON SUMAC

Poison sumac is the last of the urushiol-producing plants that we will discuss. This plant is found in the Eastern United States and typically located more in wet environments, such as around ponds and creeks. It grows as shrubs or small trees and can be identified by the red stems and multiple leaves, along with gray berries and greenish-yellow flowers. As with poison ivy and oak, exposure leads to a red blistering rash and irritation of the skin. Treatment methods are the same as poison ivy and oak.

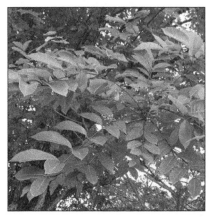 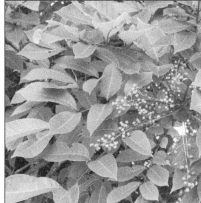

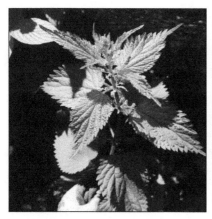
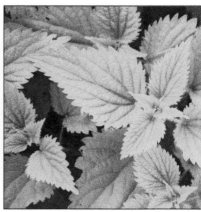

STINGING NETTLE

If you've ever been around a farm, you've probably come across some patches of stinging nettle. It grows all over North America and Europe, as well as parts of Asia and North Africa. You'll find it around farmland and streams and anywhere the ground has been disturbed. I can personally attest to the fact that it's prevalent among a lot of the southern sections of the Appalachian Trail. It's one of the larger dangerous plants, growing anywhere from 6 to 8 feet tall. The stems are most often green, but can be purple as well. The stem and leaves have stinging hairs on them that, when encountered, can cause a painful sting, followed by a localized burning and itching that can last for hours. Localized hives are possible as well.

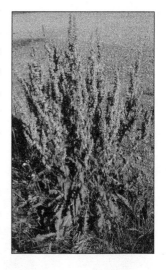

To counter the effects of stinging nettle, one can apply any variety of store-bought anti-itch creams, as well as home made remedies such as dock (shown on right), which often grows next to stinging nettle.

Oddly enough, stinging nettle itself can have medicinal properties. It's been used for food or made into tea and has long been regarded as a folk remedy for ailments such as allergies, joint pain, eczema, arthritis, gout, and anemia. Cooking the plant neutralizes its stinging properties. It is nutritious and makes great cordage. It is one of Nicole's favorite plants. "I even grow it in my garden," says Nicole.

WOOD NETTLE

Wood Nettle is the less-extreme cousin of stinging nettle. It is typically found in patches near moist areas of woodland. It stands anywhere from 2 to 4 feet tall and has green stems covered with stiff white hairs. It blooms in the summertime and produces strands of white flowers. The plant is popular with wildlife, as it provides cover for them. It also serves as a host for numerous insects and butterflies.

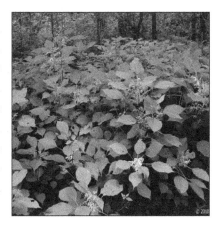

As with stinging nettle, contact with wood nettle produces a localized rash that may burn and itch. Fortunately, simply washing it off with water can greatly reduce the irritation, which usually subsides within an hour. Wood nettle can also be used for food, as some people steam it as they would any other green vegetable.

RAGWEED

The enemy of allergy sufferers throughout the entire United States, Ragweed is best known for its innate ability to cause seasonal allergy issues during late summer and throughout the fall. I've often thought that ragweed is somehow in bed with the facial tissue industry, as this one plant alone likely sells a billion boxes of tissues annually.

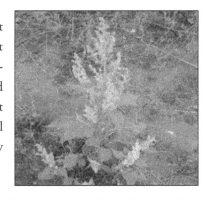

The plant itself is mostly green in color and the flowers grow from the top of the plant and elongate throughout the summer months. And as if the allergy factor alone isn't enough to hate this plant, it can also cause a rash on people who are allergic to the pollen. This can take the form of itchy patches on the skin, along with the familiar red, watery eyes and swollen eyelids. Since it can spread its pollen by contact and by airborne delivery, ragweed is likely the second most hated plant, falling only slightly behind poison ivy.

Conventional treatments include over the counter antihistamines such as Benadryl and can also be treated by natural remedies. For instance, when taken internally, stinging nettle tincture often helps ragweed sufferers as does eating local raw honey daily.

GIANT HOGWEED

I will admit that this one is new to me. During the research for this book, I learned about this plant, and if ever there was a mutant plant that a movie should be made about, it's giant hogweed. Native to central Asia, and now considered an invasive plant species in both North America and Europe, this plant can grow up to an astounding 14 feet in height (see below photos). In the United States, it is found mainly in the northeast and northwest corners of the country, but it's habitat has started to expand in recent years. It was originally introduced into Great Britain in the 19th century as an ornamental plant. The stems are greenish purple and covered with coarse, white hair. The stems produce leaves that can grow up to 5 feet across and the broad white flowers can be over 2 feet across.

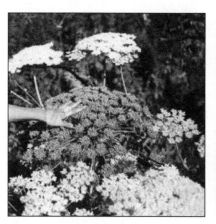 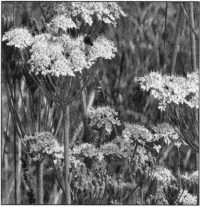

Like poison ivy, exposure to the sap of giant hogweed can cause serious skin and eye irritation, to include blistering and scarring. The rash itself resembles a burn, and can leave a long-lasting scar that is sensitive to sunlight. In addition, blindness has even been reported should it get into the eyes.

The sap itself is referred to as "phototoxic", meaning it has to be exposed to ultraviolet light in order to spur the reaction. This means it is imperative to keep any suspected exposed area away from direct sunlight for up to 2 days, while washing the area thoroughly with soap and cold water. If exposed to the eyes, flush with cold water immediately and wear sunglasses as a precaution for several days. A visit to your physician should be scheduled immediately should you begin to show signs of a reaction. This invasive plant is so hazardous that in many states, any discovery of giant hogweed mandates that the local or state environmental agencies get involved in the removal and disposal of it.

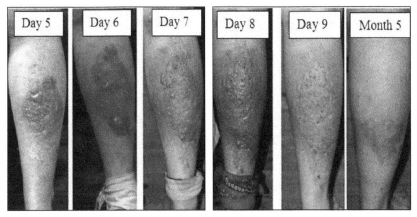

RASH DEVELOPED FROM GIANT HOGWEED EXPOSURE

WILD PARSNIP

Like giant hogweed, wild parsnip is an invasive weed species that has literally taken up roots in North America. It can be found throughout most of the country with the exception of the deep southeast. It too grows in disturbed areas and tends to spread rather quickly. It can also be found in open fields and even suburban lawns. The plant itself can grow up to 5 feet in height and has yellowish green leaves that resemble those of celery. They are coarsely toothed and usually contain around 4 or 5 leaflets. During the early summer, the weed will produce yellow flowers in small clusters.

The danger of wild parsnip is very similar to that of giant hogweed. The sap of the weed contains chemicals called furanocoumarins, which increase the skin's vulnerability to ultraviolet light. If the sap comes into contact with bare skin and is exposed to sufficient UV light, a burn will likely develop within the next 24-48 hours. This condition is referred to as photodermatitis. In some cases, it can be quite painful and severe and can result in long term or permanent discoloration of the affected site, along with an increased sensitivity to sunlight that can last for many years.

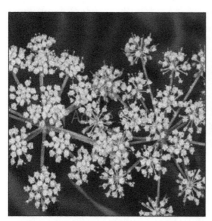 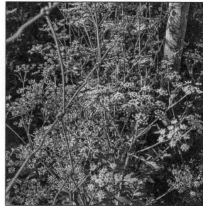

Treatment is similar to that of giant hogweed. The affected area should be covered to prevent the reaction until the skin can be thoroughly washed with soap and water. Ensure that all clothes worn in the area are completely washed separately from your other laundry. If a burn reaction does occur, consult a physician immediately to reduce the duration of the discomfort. It should be noted that this weed can be easily confused with cow parsnip, which can also cause a skin reaction upon exposure, yet is totally edible.

While not an exhaustive list, these are the primary plants that you will want to avoid while in the wilderness. If you have the chance to apply any preventative layers or creams, it would be prudent to do so. Encounters with these plants can also make a bad situation even worse. For instance, I've seen first hand the results of a fellow hiker who drank untreated water from a stream and then caught a bad case of giardia, causing him to have to stop and suffer its wrath in what he thought was a grassy patch behind some trees. It turned out that he was squatting in (you guessed it!) a giant patch of poison ivy. There were times when we thought he may have to be medevaced out due to dehydration and the extreme rash he developed. He wound up making it through the duration of the trip, but it took him several weeks afterwards to return to normal health.

A FINAL NOTE ON PLANTS

It should be noted that changing global climates are having an effect on the ecological system as a whole. Native species are, in some cases, expanding their ranges far beyond where they are traditionally found. With invasive species, some are finding it easy to expand their foothold in regions where only a few years ago, they were relatively unheard of, such as the giant hogweed. This invasive species is thriving in many areas of the country, as local and state environmental agencies are having to highlight their danger to both humans and animals. Coordinated efforts will have to be made to ensure that these invasive species' growth is halted and then eradicated in order to guarantee that native plants and animals continue to thrive in their home regions.

CHAPTER THREE

INFURIATING INSECTS

Unless you are in the dead of winter, any outdoor activity will involve the often unwanted presence of insects, both flying and crawling. While most of these critters don't harm us, there are several that can cause injuries ranging from annoying to life-threatening. The focus on this chapter will be on those biting or stinging insects which are most likely to be encountered when in the great outdoors, and what you can do to treat the wounds while in the field and at home. If you have an extreme allergy, carrying an Epipen is an excellent idea. Most people with known allergic sensitivity to insects carry an Epipen, which they inject into themselves as soon as possible after the bite or sting. This medication slows the effects of the venom in the body. Fortunately, most encounters that end with a bite or sting are non-life threatening and relatively short in duration.

ANTS

Nearly all of us are accustomed to seeing ants and the hills they build. They are crafty insects, capable of detecting food from some ways off. My family and I recently returned from a trip to Florida and brought back a dozen donuts from a world-renowned donut shop. I couldn't wait to have one for breakfast the next day. Unfortunately for me, the

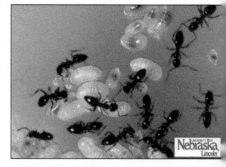

ants found them first. I've never hated a group of creatures with the fervent, white-hot rage that I felt towards those ants. Here in north Georgia, I routinely manage to mow over their hard-to-see anthills in my yard, resulting in a flood of tiny little demons erupting from the mound and onto the top of my feet. What results is an embarrassing dance of sorts to brush them off of my feet and legs. Invariably, I wind up with a dozen or so bites, and the subsequent week of itching and scratching that follows.

Believe it or not, there are actually over one thousand species of ants in the United States alone. As if that isn't disturbing enough, other countries fare even worse with several thousand different species crawling about. Fortunately, out of all those varieties, only a few pose a real threat to humans in the form of biting and stinging. Some ants bite with their mandibles and as they pinch your skin, inject a small amount of venom. Other ants sting, using their gasters, which are basically the pointy end of their abdomen. These stingers inject venom just like the biting ants. And, just so we would dislike them even more, some ants possess the ability to both bite and sting. Here in the United States, we have only a few to worry about.

ACROBAT ANTS

Named for their ability to raise their abdomens when alarmed, acrobat ants are typically not aggressive, but can turn hostile when threatened. Their coloring can range from yellowish brown to solid black and sometimes a mixture of colors. They are found mainly in the southeastern United States, primarily in Florida. Average size is around

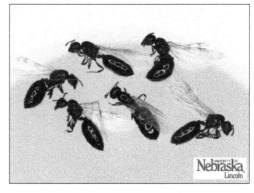

⅛ inch with queens growing the largest at around ⅜ inch. Contact with them can result in a bite or sting, or if you're truly unlucky, both. To add insult to injury, they also release a foul odor in the bite area.

CARPENTER ANTS

Aptly named for their mandibles that can pierce wood, carpenter ants are definitely biters. They are found all over the continental United States and can be a variety of colors, such as red, yellow, black, and orange. They live inside wood, specifically seeking out nests abandoned by termites. The workers

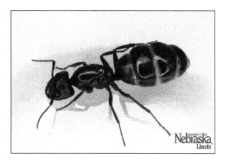

are typically around ⅜ inch long, but the winged queens can grow up to an inch long. When threatened, they don't just bite you. They inject formic acid into the bite wound, which causes moderate to severe localized pain.

PAVEMENT ANTS

These ants are your common household pests that you might find crawling on your counter or floors in search of any morsel of food. They are found mainly east of the Mississippi River, but are also encountered in the midwest. Coloration is typically brownish black and size is typically in the ⅛ inch range. As with other species,

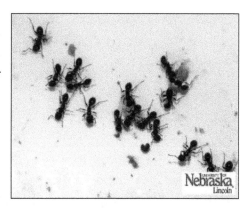

they will both bite and sting if threatened. This type of ant is known to be aggressive enough to take over neighboring colonies if they are too close.

FIRE ANTS

These guys are the ones to avoid. They are found mainly in the southeastern United States, but have been reported as far west as California. They are relatively small, averaging around ¼ inch long or less. Typically they are red in color, although some variants can have black coloring as well.

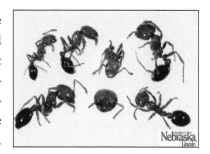

With strong mandibles and a stinger on their backside, they latch on and hit you with a one-two punch. Their sting is the most intense of all the ants you will encounter. The venom produces a severe burning sensation, with resulting swelling and blistering. Treatment is recommended immediately after exposure.

TREATMENT FOR ANT BITES AND STINGS

The majority of ant bites are not severe in nature. The discomfort at the bite location can be mitigated by washing the area with soap and water and then applying a topical anti-itch medication as needed. Rubbing salt or aloe vera can aid in the healing process as well. The itching and swelling typically disappear within a few hours or, at the longest, a few days. However, if someone is allergic to the venom or has other preexisting health conditions, the bites or stings can be much more serious. Allergic reactions can range from swelling and welts at the site of the wound, all the way up to anaphylactic shock, which is a serious condition that must be dealt with immediately.

BEES

Most readers will know what a bee looks like. If you are like me, you might have had neighbors who kept beehives to collect the honey. In the United States alone, there are upwards of 4000 species of bees. The ones we are most likely to encounter while in the outdoors that pose a threat to us are shown below.

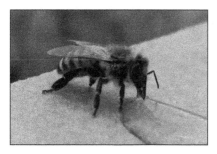 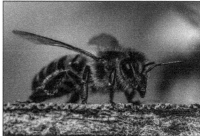

HONEY BEE

The honey bee is found throughout the continental United States in both wild and domesticated forms. They prefer more temperate environments, as some varieties do not tolerate colder weather very well. Often raised in artificial colonies, they are known by their distinct gold and brown or black bands. Size is typically around an inch long. The worker bees will sting in order to defend the colony. The stinger is barbed, and is left behind along with some of the internal organs and muscles. They are the only type of bee that die after stinging.

AFRICAN BEE

The African Bee can be found mainly in the southwest United States, although they are becoming more common in the coastal areas of the southeast as well. Their coloring is similar to the common Honey Bee, but the African Bee is usually smaller, coming in around ½ inch in length. Agitated or threatened, they have been known to chase people for more than a quarter mile in order to sting. This aggressive reputation has earned them the nickname of "killer bees."

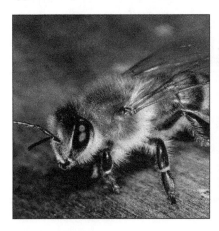 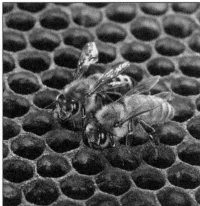

BUMBLE BEE

While encountered in most parts of the United States, the Bumble Bee is mainly native to the eastern United States and certain areas of the southwest. They are known for their distinctive yellow and black bands and can range in size from ¾ inch all the way up to 1.5 inches. They are typically peaceful, but will sting if they are threatened or the hive is disturbed.

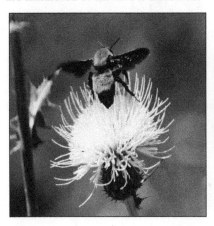 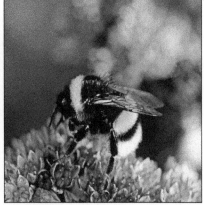

Thankfully, most of the other species do not present a threat to humans, with the exception of the carpenter bee, which can cause property damage due to its tendency to burrow into wood.

Since bees are more concerned with making honey and the pollination process, encounters with humans are usually the result of getting too close to the hive or disturbing one during its work. Hives can be found in numerous locations, such as inside dead trees, inside the walls of old houses, old boxes, and anywhere else they can find a place to build undisturbed. Domesticated bees are kept in wooden boxes where the honeycombs can be removed on a regular basis. Bees will vigorously protect both the queen and the hive, and will attack en masse when the hive is threatened. Even domestic beekeepers must wear protective clothing in order to perform their tasks without being stung.

TREATMENT FOR BEE STINGS

Fortunately, a single bee sting is not a major ordeal, unless the victim is allergic to the venom, in which case an Epipen may be required in order to stabilize the victim. In most cases, once the stinger is removed, the victim will experience painful swelling at the site of the injection, which can last several days. Treatments normally consist of topical medications that reduce the swelling and burning sensation. In the field, chewed-up plantain leaf is a great way to stop the bite or sting. Application of baking soda and water or apple cider vinegar can be applied to the site of the sting and will help in the healing process as well. In the event that someone encounters a swarm of bees and is stung multiple times, the outcome may be much more serious, with hospitalization required if they have a sensitivity to bee venom. Nicole uses a blend of plantain and calendula to stop the sting (see appendix for the recipe).

It should be noted that one should never try to eradicate a colony of bees on their own. To do so is to risk serious injury. Beekeepers can often be contacted to come remove a colony in its entirety, transporting them to an area where they can continue to benefit the environment without encountering humans.

WASPS

If you are anything like me, your first recollection of wasps may have something to do with your father spraying a massive nest up in some obscure corner of the outside of your house and then running away to avoid the angry mob. Growing up in the south, it felt like wasps reproduced even quicker than rabbits, and there was always another nest popping up somewhere. Like the other stinging insects we have discussed, there 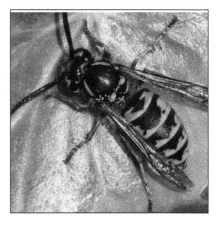 are upwards of 4,000 species of wasps in North America alone. Fortunately, only a handful of these species are trouble-makers.

HORNETS

I had no idea that these guys were members of the wasp species until I began researching information for this book. These are the big, ugly creatures that no one wants to encounter. My earliest memory of a hornet was when I was around 7 years old. My father had told me to go put some shoes on and not walk around my grandfather's yard barefooted. Of course, in my 7 year old wisdom, I immediately disregarded his advice. The 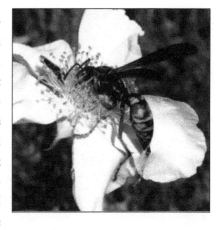 result? I stepped right on a hornet and was promptly stung between my big toe and the next. The pain was intense, and the tears flowed immediately. My foot and ankle swelled to the point that my parents were worried that I would have to go to the doctor. After a few days, the swelling began to subside, but the pain lasted several days beyond that.

The most commonly-encountered hornets in North America are shown below.

BALD-FACED HORNET

The Bald-faced Hornet is found in all 50 states. They are distinguishable by their white and black coloring. Size ranges from ½ inch for workers to over an inch for queens. They build nests in all types of environments from residential settings to forests and meadows. Their nests are above ground, such as on a tree limb or an outcropping on a house. The nest itself is gray in color and resembles a pear or sphere-shaped mass made out of paper with an opening at the bottom. They are extremely protective of their nests and will sting repeatedly if they feel threatened. They are also known to kill other insects such as flies and yellow jackets and feed their chewed-up bodies to their larvae.

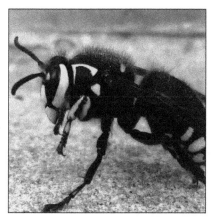 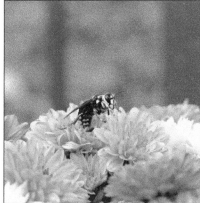

EUROPEAN HORNET

The European Hornet is also referred to as the giant hornet or the brown hornet. Their color scheme is typically a yellow and black lower body with reddish brown upper body and head. It's size ranges from ¾ inch up to 1.5 inches, and it's the only true hornet native to the United States. Their habitat is from the northeastern United States out to the Dakotas, and as far south as Louisiana and Florida. Like the Bald-faced Hornet, the European Hornet will build paper-like nests in trees and along buildings, but will also build inside walls and sometimes at ground level in rocky environments. They are extremely aggressive and will deliver a painful sting if provoked. Unlike most members of the wasp family, the European Hornet is known to be active at night.

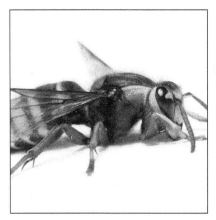 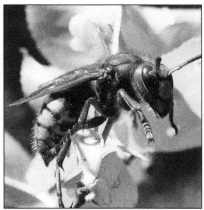

It's easy to see why hornets are feared by most people. Their aggressive nature and powerful sting makes them a formidable opponent. I recall the time my aunt was stung by a hornet from an unnoticed nest in the small tree next to where she parked her car. Without saying a word, she walked inside, returned with a wad of newspaper, some lighter fluid, and a box of matches. She proceeded to douse the newspaper in the lighter fluid, roll it up as tight as possible, and crammed it into the opening of the nest and lit it on fire, while dousing the nest as well. As you can imagine, the results were lethal. A few hearty souls escaped their burning death trap, but the majority were taken out. Being a teenager at the time, I can remember debating that it was either the coolest or the dumbest course of action that I had ever seen. To put it mildly, as with bee colonies, it's best to let a professional deal with a nest especially if it's in close proximity to your home.

TREATMENT FOR HORNET STINGS

If you do find yourself stung by a hornet, the same treatment as bee stings applies. An over-the-counter or homemade topical treatment will reduce the swelling and throbbing pain and, in the field, applying chewed-up plantain leaf will relieve the pain. An ice pack can give relief as well. If allergies to the venom are present, an Epipen may be required.

PAPER WASPS

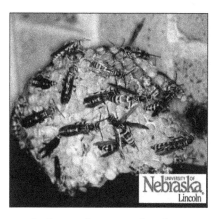

These guys are the ones that build the wonderful little nests up in the corners of your house with the little white pods in them. They will also build anywhere they can find adequate cover. I've found nests in my shed, my boat, the lid to my propane tank, etc. In the wild, be cautious of brush piles, fallen trees, or anywhere else that may provide a cozy nest-building area. They are creative, so ensure that you know what might be present before sticking your hand into an area you can't see very well. Coloration can range from yellow and black to reddish brown. Size is ½ inch up to 1.5 inches. There are over 20 species in North America alone.

They typically will leave you alone unless you are near a nest, in which case they will deliver a painful sting. Thankfully, treatment is the same as bees and hornets, with minor pain and swelling being the most common reaction. Nests are typically dealt with using aerosol sprays that can be applied from a distance, and most effectively in the evening, when the concentration of wasps is the highest. Just be ready to move should the swarm begin to come at you.

YELLOWJACKETS

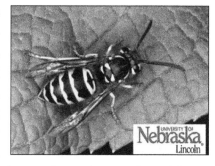

These guys, although small in size, can pack a major punch. Instantly recognizable by their black and yellow coloring, these wasps are most commonly build their nests in burrows in the ground, although they are also known to build in walls and other confined spaces. They are found throughout the continental United States, but are particularly abundant in the southeastern United States. They are typically in the ½ to ¾ inch size range.

They are my second least favorite stinging insect, as I spent several years running a lawn service and routinely encountered them as they would come boiling out of the ground after being mowed over or walked near. These guys find strength in numbers, and the situation can get serious in a hurry. It's not uncommon to be stung multiple times as they swarm out of the nest and attack.

TREATMENT FOR YELLOWJACKETS:

As with the other wasp species, the severity of the sting will dictate the treatment. A solitary sting, while painful, will usually subside after an application of a topical ointment or salve, plantain leaf, or a simple cold pack. Multiple stings may require an Epipen or even hospitalization. If encountering a nest, the best course of action is to simply vacate the area. Trying to swat or kill yellow jackets will simply make the situation worse, as they release a hormone when crushed that attracts others to the area. Also, they love to be around sweet-smelling and tasting food and drink. This is why they are commonly encountered as we try to enjoy a backyard cookout or a picnic by the lake.

If you do happen to find a nest around your property, take care in the way that you dispatch it. I'm sure we've all seen the "soak the hole with gas and light a match while running away" method. While certainly effective (and oftentimes comical), this is also a wonderful way to set your yard or property on fire, especially if conditions are dry. There are many products available to eradicate them, and, if you simply must use gasoline, just pour it in the whole and resist the urge to light it. The fumes alone will kill the majority and the survivors will seek another location in which to build. The best time to apply any kind of treatment is at night, when the whole colony is present in the nest.

MOSQUITOS

These guys need no introduction. Found through-out the continental United States, mosquitoes ha-rass those of us who enjoy the outdoors in all seasons except late fall and winter time. While the bite itself rarely causes much discomfort except for an annoying itch, the insects themselves transfer diseases such as West Nile virus and encephalitis. Averaging around ½ inch in size, they bring a level of annoyance that is much larger.

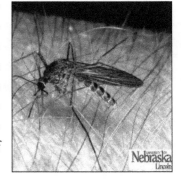

TREATMENT FOR MOSQUITO BITES

Treatment for the bites can be as simple as washing with cold water or applying a dab of topical ointment (see appendix) or applying a chewed-up plantain leaf (really!). The key to dealing with mosquitos is prevention. They are found in the highest numbers in areas that are damp, such as around bodies of water or swamps. They are typically at their worst during the late spring and summer, and can turn an outdoor gathering into a miserable experience. Fortunately, sprays and yard treatments are available to minimize the chances of being pestered by these flying annoyances. However, do your homework before spraying or applying, as some brands contain chemicals such as DEET that have been shown to be harmful to humans and pets. Treating your clothing with Permethrin is a good way to deter mosquitoes as is a natural spray you can make at home (see appendix).

CATERPILLARS

Most people think of caterpillars as cute little bugs that build a cocoon and emerge as a beautiful, colorful butterfly. As with other species of insects that we have discussed, there are many different species of caterpillars. Fortunately, only a handful pose a threat to humans. Unfortunately, that handful can certainly pack a punch when it comes to their sting. Here are the species to avoid:

SADDLEBACK CATERPILLAR

This brightly-colored guy is definitely unique, and the name certainly makes sense. Found primarily in the eastern United States, they range in size from 1 to 1.75 inches. They are certainly beautiful to observe, but do not attempt to pick them up. The horn-like appendages 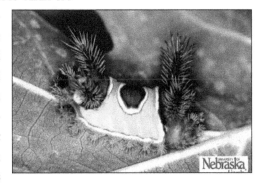 on both ends of his body are actually barbed spines that will stick in your skin and break off, allowing poison to spill onto your skin. The result is localized swelling along with a rash that can be quite painful. Individuals with sensitive skin or other topical skin issues may even need to seek professional medical help.

HAG MOTH CATERPILLAR

Also referred to as the "monkey slug", this caterpillar appears to have tentacles similar to that of a starfish. Rather than barbs at each end of its body, as in the case of the saddleback, the monkey slug is covered with barb-like hairs over its entire body and has a similar reaction to being picked up and handled. Their habitat is from the midwest to the east coast and they range from 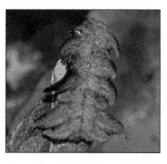 ¾ to 1 inch in length. Coloration is typically shades of brown, although black, white, and tan variations are also encountered. Their sting is similar in severity to the saddleback, so it's best just to avoid these guys as well.

PUSS CATERPILLAR

While researching insects for this book, I came upon one site that aptly described this caterpillar as resembling a tribble from the Star Trek television series (the younger generations may have to Google this). Their range is from New Jersey to Florida, and as far west as Arkansas and Texas. Their color scheme is typically rust-colored or 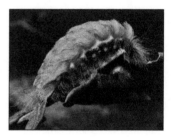 mustard brown with some black coloration often present as well. As cute and fluffy as they might appear, these guys are the ones to avoid the most. They are only about an inch long, but the sting from their barbs has been described as "excruciating" and "agonizing" as well as "long-lasting."

STINGING ROSE CATERPILLAR

These yellowish-brown caterpillars have a distinctive pinstripe color scheme down their backs. They are relatively small, ranging in size from ¾ to ⅞ inches long. They are found from New York to Florida, and westward from Missouri to Texas. As with others in this section, they will sting if disturbed, resulting in a memorable experience. It's best to simply admire them from a distance.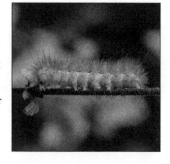

SPINY ELM CATERPILLAR

This caterpillar is easily distinguished by a black body with white spots and a line of red dots across its back. They can be up to 2 inches long when grown and are found all throughout the continental United States. Unlike many of the other caterpillars we have discussed, this variety

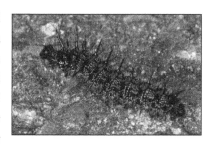

prefers to live in groups, making an encounter with them in the wild potentially more dangerous. If you see a cluster of these guys feeding on a plant, it's best just to leave them be. Multiple stings could certainly ruin a family walk in the woods.

WHITE FLANNEL CATERPILLAR

This caterpillar has a color scheme that is yellow, orange and black. They are typically around an inch in length and are found primarily in the southeastern United States. This is another example of a caterpillar that may look benign, but a few quick seconds of handling will certainly prove otherwise!

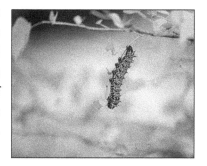

CROWNED SLUG CATERPILLAR

This interesting-looking caterpillar has its spines around the perimeter of it's flat body. These are found from Massachusetts to Florida and westward to Mississippi to Missouri and should definitely be avoided. Their color scheme is quite distinct, with a green body and reddish-yellow accents down their back and on their extremities. Size is typically around ⅝ inches.

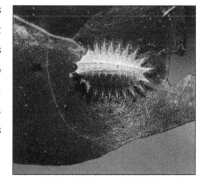

IO MOTH CATERPILLAR

This guy should be a no-brainer when it comes to picking up. Resembling a walking cactus, this caterpillar has barbs around it's entire body, each ready to deliver a painful sting. They are found primarily in the eastern United States. Their color scheme is a green body with a reddish and white stripe down their sides. They can grow up to 2.25 inches in length. This is another variety of caterpillar that can be found in groups, so

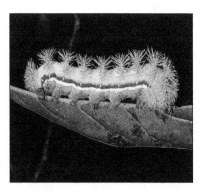

be careful that you don't accidentally grab a handful when pushing away tree limbs or walking through dense plant growth.

WHITE MARKED TUSSOCK MOTH CATERPILLAR

These caterpillars are considered a threat to both humans and trees. With its distinctive red head and black and yellow or orange stripes, this caterpillar will eat anything that is woody and large numbers can quickly decimate the area in which they occupy. Typical range is from the eastern United States to the midwest-

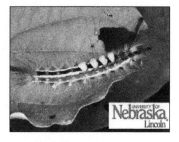

ern states. They range in size from ½ inch up to 1.4 inches in length. Their spiky tufts of hair contain chemicals that often cause an allergic reaction on human skin when contact is made, and the hairs themselves are barbed, which can make them difficult to remove. These guys are best left alone.

BUCK MOTH CATERPILLAR

Looking like a walking sea urchin, this caterpillar wears an armor of barbs all around its body. Known by its distinctive color scheme of black with white or yellowish spots, this guy sports a sting that has been known to last up to a full two weeks. They are found across all of the continental

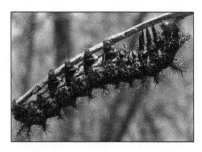

United States, and are some of the larger caterpillars, growing anywhere from 2 to 3 inches in length.

TREATMENT FOR CATERPILLARS

Since the sting from all caterpillars is similar, only differing in the degree of severity, the treatments for them are similar as well. If exposed to one, ensure that the barbs or hairs have been removed from your skin. Since some tend to stick in the top layer of skin, a piece of scotch tape or other sticky substance can help remove any remaining barbs. Afterwards, washing the affected area with cold water and soap can help with the burning sensation. Other relief can be brought about with the topical application of a mixture of baking soda and water or by using topical hydrocortisone or antihistamine creams. In cases where the sting location begins to blister, becomes worse over time, or the pain reaches levels that are no longer bearable, a trip to a doctor is probably in order so that more powerful treatment can be administered. Children, the elderly, and people with allergies and skin sensitivity should be closely monitored after a caterpillar sting to ensure that they do not suffer a severe reaction to the poison.

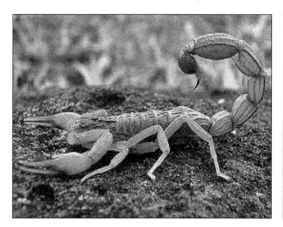 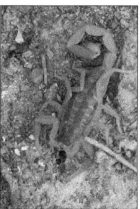

SCORPIONS

When we think about scorpions, most people likely envision the southwest region of the country. The truth of the matter is that scorpions are found throughout the United States. While there are about 1500 known species of scorpions, there are only about 75 species residing in the United States. Fortunately for us, out of the 1500 known species, only 25 have a sting that is potentially hazardous to humans. Of those 25 species, only one lives in the United States. The bark scorpion is mainly found in the American southwest, and it's sting can cause extreme pain and can endanger the lives of people with weak immune systems, such as young children and the elderly. It's size ranges from 2 to 3 inches, and their color scheme is typically a uniform tan or yellowish-brown, with some having a darker appearance on their backs.

Scorpions are nocturnal insects, so going barefoot at night isn't always the best idea if you are in an area that is home to scorpions. And just because the bark scorpion is the only known species in the US to cause major harm to its victims, that doesn't mean to let your guard down around other species, because they will sting as well. The sting may not result in hospitalization, but it is certainly painful enough to remind us to avoid them. Since they tend to favor dark areas, they are often found hiding in shoes and clothes, so it's a good idea to always shake them out before dressing.

TREATMENT FOR SCORPIONS

If stung by a scorpion, the victim will likely experience one or more of the following symptoms:

• Localized pain at the site of the sting
• Numbness and tingling in the extremities
• Blurred vision
• Slurred speech
• Facial numbness
• Muscle twitching

First aid in most cases is no more complicated than washing the affected area with soap and water and applying a cool compress to soothe the pain. Only in a minority of cases will further professional medical treatment be required. Most cases of scorpion stings just result in the victim riding it out for a few days until the pain subsides.

SPIDERS

If there is one category of insects (well, technically they are arachnids) that absolutely creeps me out, it's spiders. Nicole, on the other hand, tends to love the little critters, and rightly so, as they are an important part of the ecosystem. While they still give me the willies, I can't argue with her logic. I've been bitten several times over the course of my life and these little creatures can at times be problematic, to say the least. While there are over 3000 known species of spiders in North America, there are fortunately only four distinct species that pose a serious threat to humans. The rest are harmless and apparently draw contentment from knowing they make me scream like a teenage girl watching a horror movie.

RECLUSES

There are 11 species of recluse spiders found in North America, with the Brown Recluse being the most notable, although white, gray, and black species can also be found. The typical Brown Recluse range is from Nebraska to Ohio and then southward from Texas to Florida. They are not large spiders, typical-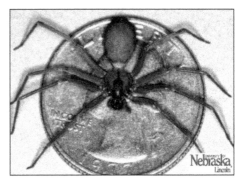ly coming in around ⅜ inches and tend to be just as happy indoors as they do outdoors, so encounters with humans are likely. Fortunately, recluses tend to only bite when they feel threatened. The effects of a bite can range from redness, swelling, and pain at the bite location, to major tissue loss and infection if left untreated. Often times, the skin around the bite location may turn a deep blue or purple and develop a red ring around it.

I worked with a lady once who was bitten at home and merely wrapped the area with gauze and medical tape after applying a topical ointment. Days later, her leg hurt to the point where she was unable to perform her job duties. When I took her off the assembly line, she pulled up her pant leg to show that the bite area had swelled up to the point that her skin was in danger of splitting and a discharge was present. I convinced her to go to her physician and seek treatment. It took several days for her to return to work. She explained that her physician told her that the bite area had become infected and all the surrounding tissue had become necrotic and he had to remove several areas of dead tissue. The wound channel went nearly to her bone. It required the wound to be packed and the bandages changed several times per day until the medication had the chance to treat the bite and allow it to begin to heal. She said the doctor told her that she wasn't far from having to be hospitalized due to the severity of the bite and the amount of time she left it untreated. It took a few months for the bite location to return to somewhat normal, and there was quite a bit of scarring where the doctor had removed dead tissue. Ironically, she never felt the spider bite her. She just noticed a spot on her leg that began to hurt and swell. The doctor was confident that it had been a Recluse bite.

WIDOWS

While there are 32 species of widows, the most commonly-encountered variety is the well-known Black Widow. Known for its distinctive black body and reddish hourglass design on its belly, this species of spider likes to hide in sheltered areas such as wood piles and storage sheds and anywhere else that will keep it out of the light.

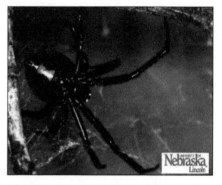

Other color variations exist, such as the red widow, brown widow and gray widow. While their typical habitat is the southeastern United States, they are also routinely encountered as far west as Texas and as far north as Ohio. They are normally around ½ inch in length. I've encountered quite a few in stacks of concrete building blocks and under the water meter cover in my front yard as well as my propane tank lid in my backyard.

These spiders have a reputation as being one of the most prolific biters due to the fact that they often react out of a defensive posture when their cover is disturbed. The venom from a widow is approximately 15 times more potent than that of a rattlesnake. The bite itself can range in severity from unnoticed to extreme pain and stiffness at the bite site. Symptoms of the bite include the standard headache, nausea and vomiting and can also include abdominal pain and cramping, hypertension, chilling, and nervous system issues. Those with weakened immune systems are particularly susceptible to the venom, but fortunately less than 1% of victims bitten by a black widow will succumb to the venom. This is mainly due to advances in antivenin availability at hospitals. Still, seek help as soon as possible!

HOBO SPIDER

These guys are usually found in the western part of the country, as they prefer dry environments. They are normally found around ground level and will happily occupy basements and crawl spaces of homes. Coloration is typically light to medium brown with darker extremities and size ranges from 1 to 1.75 inches. They can be quite aggressive and are known to bite with little or no provocation. As a matter of fact, Nicole was once bitten by one of these that was hiding in a folded blanket in a closet.

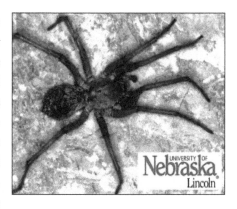

A hobo spider bite is most often painless, with a redness appearing around the bite area. Eventually, the bite will turn into an oozing blister, usually within 24 hours. Other symptoms can include nausea, weakness, fatigue, temporary memory loss, vision impairment, and severe headaches that may last several days. The bite location can take several weeks up to a few months to fully heal, as the amount of skin necrosis may vary. While the bites are rarely fatal, it's important to seek medical attention to minimize tissue damage and loss.

YELLOW SAC SPIDER

These spiders can vary in their color scheme based off what they last ate, as they are somewhat transparent. They are nocturnal hunters that have no problem taking up residence around people. Size is rather small, with most found in the ¼ to ½ inch range. They are found throughout the country and are believed to be responsible for the majority of nuisance bites in the US. Fortunately, their venom is only mildly toxic, and while they can be painful, the amount of necrosis is usually negligible and heasl quickly with a minimal amount of scarring.

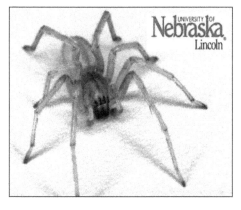

TREATMENT FOR SPIDER BITES

When it comes to first aid for spider bites, the most important thing to remember is not to panic, especially if the bite occurs or is noticed while outdoors. While the bite may be very painful, the chances of long term damage or death are negligible as long as proper treatment is obtained. If you feel you were bitten by a spider, you should wash the location with soap and water and apply a topical antibiotic ointment. A cold compress or ice pack can also be used to help reduce swelling, as well as elevating the affected limb. Over the counter medications such as ibuprofen can help alleviate the swelling and antihistamines such as Benadryl can help with any related itching. If the bite site continues to intensify in pain or size, professional medical help should be sought immediately to minimize the potential damage to the bite location.

BITING FLIES

While most people see flies as merely an annoyance, there are a few species that will inflict bites on humans. Fortunately, the likelihood of transmitting a disease to humans, while possible, is extremely rare. Unfortunately, for people with severe allergies the saliva can, in rare cases, trigger a very serious and sometimes life-threatening reaction. This is in part due to the fact that the saliva itself is an anticoagulant. Biting flies have mouth appendages that literally slice the skin open and the fly proceeds to suck up the blood that comes out of the wound. While this all sounds like something from a bad science-fiction movie, the truth for the majority of us is that a biting fly simply inflicts a painful bite that lingers for a few days. There are numerous species of biting flies, but we will only discuss the most prevalent ones that you might likely encounter.

DEER FLY

These guys are the annoying little creatures that love to buzz around your head before biting. They can be found around watery areas such as creeks and swampy land all throughout the United States. Their color scheme is usually brown or black with bands. They are most prevalent in

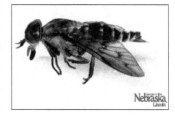

spring time and grow to about a quarter inch long. Unfortunately, these flies are one of the few types that have been known to transmit diseases to humans. On rare occasions, deer flies have been found to pass on rabbit fever (Tularemia) after coming in contact with infected animals. The bite of these flies can be painful, especially when encountering them in large numbers, and they are known to bite the same area multiple times.

HORSE FLY

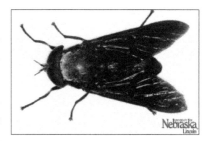

These are the larger cousin to the deer fly. Reaching sizes of an inch or longer, these flies are found around damp areas and are commonly encountered around livestock. They are present throughout the United States, with the greatest concentrations in and around Florida. Their coloration is typically a brownish-black, although solid colored varieties are not uncommon. They are aggressive, often returning to a bite two or more times to ensure that they lap up all the resulting blood. Their bite can be quite painful as well.

STABLE FLY

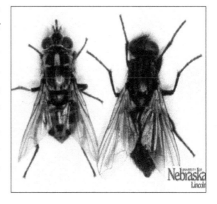

These devious little guys resemble the common house fly with the exception of a pointed appendage beneath it's head, which it uses to suck up the blood from its bites. They are found throughout the United States, mainly wherever cattle or other livestock is present. Size is small, ranging from ¼ to 5/16 inches and coloration is typically a lighter black or brown with clear wings.

These flies are most prevalent in the late summer and fall and have been known to fly several miles to find prey. While they most often target livestock, pets and people are targets of opportunity as well. They prefer to bite in the early morning or late afternoon and tend to target the ankles when inflicting their painful bites, which have been described as sharp and stabbing.

BLACK FLY

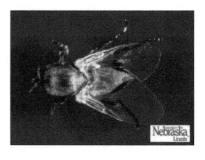

This species of flies are small in size, coming in no larger than about ⅛ of an inch. They are found throughout the United States, with the largest concentrations in the northern regions and into Canada. They tend to favor moist environments and are often encountered around creeks and rivers. In some parts of the country, they are referred to as "buffalo gnats". Coloration can range from black to various shades of yellow or gray. These guys will fly up to 10 miles in search of prey. They are most prevalent in late spring and early summer and their bites often cause considerable swelling and bleeding, and can sometimes be itchy and slow to heal. These flies target the head and anywhere else that clothing fits tightly.

GREENHEAD FLY

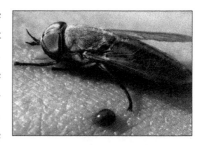

With a similar appearance to that of the Horse Fly, the Greenhead Fly sports a dark brown body with a distinctive green head. Size is usually ½ inches or larger. They are found typically in coastal marshes in the eastern United States. They are aggressive biters, using their scissor-like appendages to tear the skin, and then douse the area with a saliva that stings and burns as it stimulates blood flow, which the fly sucks up with a straw-like appendage. They seem to be particularly troublesome in mid to late summer time and will often be unfazed by all but the strongest bug repellant.

BITING MIDGE

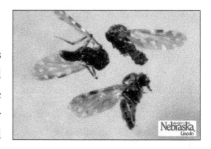

This type of fly is the smallest that one is likely to encounter. They are dark-bodied with light-colored wings and at no more than 1/32 of an inch long, they also go by nicknames such as "punkies", "gnats", and my personal favorite, "no-see-ums". Their miniscule size allows them to find their way into any type of dwelling. They are most prevalent around the shores of lakes and ponds and around beaches and are encountered nationwide. I was in Savannah in early 2018 with my son on a fishing trip, and the biting midges ran us off from more than one secluded fishing location. As luck would have it, I ran out of bug spray, and they took full advantage of the situation. On numerous occasions, I would slap one and find a trickle of blood running down my arm or leg. While most species target humans exclusively, some will actually suck the blood of other insects, including mosquitoes, spreading any diseases they may have been carrying.

TREATMENT FOR BITING FLIES

When it comes to first aid for biting fly bites, the treatment is much the same as for other insect stings. Washing the wound with soap and water to avoid infection is the first step. Applying a topical antibiotic ointment and then a bandage should follow. The bite location will sometimes itch and swell, so a topical antihistamine lotion may be in order. The bite will usually heal within a few days, but if the pain persists, or the swelling continues, you may be having an allergic reaction and should likely see a physician. If outdoors, a suitable bug repellant will definitely help. If you don't like the harsh chemicals that are often found in store-bought sprays, you can make your own at home. I found many recipes online, most of which consisted of mixing a pint of white vinegar with a few ounces of baby oil and some dish soap mixed in a spray bottle. To give the mixture a little added kick, add in 5-10 drops of eucalyptus or tea tree oil. These essential oils seem to be quite effective at repelling biting flies. A few drops of citronella oil will help keep the mosquitos away as well.

TICKS

If you have spent any time at all in the great outdoors, you likely have discovered a tick attached to you somewhere. Dog owners know all too well the struggle of keeping them off your pets, especially during the summer months. Most of the time they can be safely removed and there is little evidence that you ever had an issue. However, ticks do transmit disease, so it is important to know what species of ticks are in your area of the country. In this section we will review the most common species throughout North America and when they are most active. Like spiders, ticks are in the arachnid family. They are typically around 0.1 to 0.3 inches in length when unfed, expanding to up to 0.5 inches or longer after feeding. Colorations shown in the accompanying pics show what the average of the species looks like, but that can vary with different sub-species, so be aware of what types of ticks are in your region and what their particular color schemes are.

AMERICAN DOG TICK

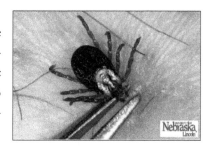

Also referred to as wood ticks, these ticks are found east of the Rocky Mountains and in some areas along the Pacific Coast. This species of tick is known to transmit Tularemia and Rocky Mountain Spotted Fever.

Tularemia is characterized by symptoms ranging from skin ulcers at the bite site, swelling of regional lymph glands, and a sore throat. More serious forms of the disease will include cough, chest pain, difficulty breathing and fevers that can go as high as 104 degrees. While the disease can be life-threatening, most cases can be treated by a course of antibiotics. Rocky Mountain Spotted Fever is a bacterial disease that can exhibit symptoms such as fevers, headaches, and rashes. It can be deadly if not addressed early with the proper course of antibiotics.

The highest risk of being bitten by the American Dog Tick comes in the spring and summer. The female of the species is the most likely to bite a human.

BLACKLEGGED TICK

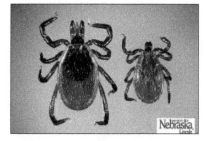

Also referred to as deer ticks, these ticks are most commonly encountered across the eastern United States. These ticks can transmit a variety of diseases, the most common and serious of which is Lyme Disease. Symptoms vary based on the timing of the bite. Early symptoms will show up anywhere from 3 to 30 days after the initial bite. They include fever, chills, headaches, fatigue, aching in the joints and muscles and swelling of the lymph nodes. In addition, a rash may begin at the site of the bite and gradually expand over the following days sometimes reaching 12 inches in diameter or more. The bite may feel warm to the touch but is typically not painful or itchy, but may take on the look of a bull's eye as it spreads. The rash can, in some cases, show up on any part of the body. After removing the tick, save it if possible to be tested for Lyme Disease.

Later symptoms can show up months after the initial bite and are more serious. They include severe headaches, stiffness of the neck, additional rashes, arthritis with associated joint pain and swelling concentrated in the knees and other large joints, facial palsy, heart palpitations, episodes of dizziness, shortness of breath, nerve pain, numbness, tingling in the extremities, inflammation of the brain and spinal cord, and problems with short-term memory. If you have any of these symptoms after experiencing a tick bite, seek medical attention immediately. Lyme Disease is often treated quickly with antibiotics if caught early, but if treatment is delayed, the treatment regimen can be much longer and more involved. Teasel root (Dipsacus sylvestris) is known to help pull the Lyme-causing spirochaete from your tissues, exposing it to your immune system for eradication.

The Blacklegged Tick is most likely to bite during any season except winter. The female of the species is the most likely to bite a human.

BROWN DOG TICK

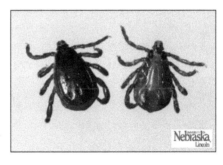

This species of tick is found nationwide. They are known to transmit Rocky Mountain spotted fever, primarily in the southwestern United States and along the southern border. This disease is quite serious. Early symptoms include the standard fever, headache, nausea, stomach issues, muscle pain, and lack of appetite. Within two to four days after symptoms appear, a rash will develop throughout the body. Treatment for Rocky Mountain spotted fever is accomplished through the antibiotic doxycycline. Even after treatment, some patients are left with permanent damage. This can include amputation of limbs or digits, hearing loss, paralysis, and mental disability. These type of ticks are most commonly found on dogs, but will bite humans or other mammals given the opportunity.

GULF COAST TICK

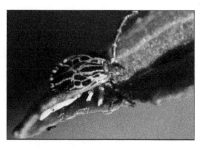

This species of tick is found mostly around the Atlantic coast area in the southeastern United States. They are known to transmit R. parkeri, which is a form of spotted fever. The first symptom to manifest with this fever is a dark scab at the site of the bite, which develop a few days after the bite is inflicted. Additional symptoms include fever, headache, rashes, and muscle aches. Treatment for this condition typically includes the antibiotic doxycycline. This type of tick is most commonly found on deer and other wildlife, but will bite humans when given the opportunity.

LONE STAR TICK

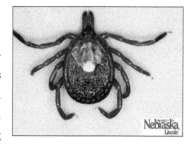

The Lone Star Tick is recognized by the single white dot on the back of the female. As you can likely guess by its name, it is found widely among the southeastern United States. They are associated with transmitting ehrlichiosis, Heartland virus, tularemia, and STARI. Since each of these diseases can be deadly, we will take a brief look at the symptoms and treatment options for each. We discussed tularemia in the American Dog Tick section.

Ehrlichiosis typically begins to manifest itself between one and two weeks after being bitten by an infected tick. Symptoms include a combination of fever, headache, chills, fatigue, muscle pain, gastrointestinal problems, confusion, red eyes, and rashes on the body. Treatment for this condition is mainly accomplished through the administration of the antibiotic doxycycline.

Heartland virus is a serious condition that, as of this time, has no known treatment. Most people suffering from it experience similar symptoms as other tick-borne illnesses. The incubation period can be around two weeks and eventually manifests itself in the form of fever, fatigue, decreased appetite, headache, nausea, diarrhea, and various muscle or joint aches. All known patients who have contacted the virus have required hospitalization, although most recovered fully. Unfortunately, there have been a few deaths associated with the virus.

STARI is typically diagnosed within seven days of a bite from an infected tick. The most visible symptom is a rash that starts small and then expands outward. Other symptoms include fatigue, headache, fever, and muscle pain. There is no specific treatment for STARI, but since it so closely resembles the symptoms of Lyme disease, most doctors will treat patients with a series of oral antibiotics.

Lone Star ticks also have a saliva that can be irritating to the skin. Redness and discomfort at the bite site is common. This is a species of tick that is considered very aggressive and will commonly bite humans.

ROCKY MOUNTAIN WOOD TICK

This type of tick is found in the Rocky Mountain states and up into Canada. It favors elevations from 4,000 up to 10,000 feet. In addition to Rocky Mountain spotted fever and Tularemia, the Rocky Mountain Wood Tick is also a transmitter of Colorado tick fever. This tick-borne illness is characterized by fever, chills, head and 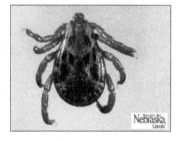 body aches, and an overall feeling of fatigue. Currently, there are no medications or vaccines to treat this disease. While most patients recover over time, consult a physician if you feel that you may have the disease. This type of tick typically feeds on large mammals, so they have no problem whatsoever biting a human.

WESTERN BLACKLEGGED TICK

These ticks are found along the Pacific coastline of the US, mainly in California. In addition to transmitting Lyme disease, these ticks also are known to carry Anaplasmosis. This disease starts out similar to most tick-borne illnesses and includes fever, chills, muscle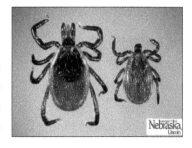

aches, nausea, vomiting, and diarrhea. If not treated in time, symptoms become more severe. They include respiratory failure, bleeding, organ failure, and in some cases, can result in death. Thankfully, if caught in time and treated with doxycycline, the patient normally recovers. It's typically the female of the species that bite humans.

PREVENTION MEASURES & TREATMENT FOR TICK BITES

As you can see, ticks are a potentially dangerous insect to come into contact with. While the diseases discussed here are serious in nature, most bites do not result in a serious illness. However, since the possibility does exist, precautions should be taken when outdoors in an area where ticks are common. If you have pets, especially dogs, make sure they are treated monthly with a tick preventative. This will help to ensure that they do not bring any ticks into the home.

Clothing should be tucked in wherever possible, such as pant legs tucked into boots and the wearing of long sleeves. Tick repellent should be worn on any exposed skin (see appendix for a natural repellent recipe). When returning home, it's advisable to check oneself for ticks, as they are often quite difficult to see without a deliberate examination. If one is found, it's best to use a pair of tweezers and pull it out slowly while gripping it as close to the head as possible. Dispose of it by flushing it down the toilet or save it for testing if you think it may be a Lyme disease-causing tick. Note the location and time of the bite and monitor it for any changes, such as swelling, itching, and the symptoms discussed above. If any of these begin to develop, it would be advisable to visit a physician to be checked out professionally as soon as possible. With symptoms sometimes showing up weeks after the initial bite, it's important to begin treatment as soon as possible in order to minimize the duration of the disease.

MISCELLANEOUS OTHER SPECIES

CENTIPEDES

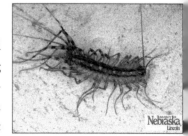

These interesting creatures are most often found in moist, dark, protected areas, such as in rotting logs and leaves and under rocks. They are encountered throughout the United States and range in size from around an inch to over a foot. The most common variety is the house centipede. Nicole recently encountered one in the tropics that was 8" long and hiding in a shoe.

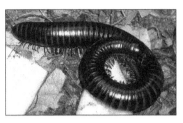

They are often confused with millipedes (as seen on the right), with the main difference being that centipedes have one pair of legs per body segment, while millipedes have two pairs. Centipedes also move much faster than milli-pedes when disturbed. While creepy, millipedes pose no threat to humans. Their main defense mechanism when disturbed or picked up is to secrete a pungent liquid and curl its body up. Centipedes, on the other hand, do pose a slight threat to humans.

TREATMENT FOR CENTIPEDE BITES

Since they are carnivorous in nature, they kill their prey by injecting them with venom from the modified legs on their first segment. The bite site typically shows two puncture wounds. Fortunately, the dosage that they dispense when biting a human is not sufficient to produce anything more than a sharp pain and resulting localized swelling. Most bites require nothing more than a thorough cleaning and a local anesthetic to provide pain relief. In some rare cases, however, the bite can cause more serious symptoms. This most often is found in young children and the elderly, and people with allergies that react with the venom. Symptoms here can include intense itching, headache, swollen lymph nodes, dizziness, nausea, heart palpitations, anxiety, and elevated blood pressure. In the most extreme cases, local-ized tissue damage may occur. For patients exhibiting these symptoms, professional medical care is advised, where antihistamine and occasionally powerful narcotics are required for treatment. Since centipedes rarely bite unprovoked, it's best to leave them alone when you come across them in the outdoors. If you are finding an abun-dance of them in your home, you may want to consult a pest control company.

LEECHES

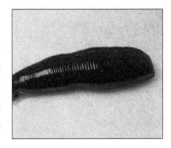

Leeches are a common occurrence around most creeks and other bodies of water. North America hosts 79 species of leeches and size can range from a few inches to nearly a foot. Wading around while fishing or crossing from one side to another will often result in picking up one of these hitchhikers, usually around the feet. As a kid, I often spent long days wading through the creek near my house fishing for bream and redeye bass. When leaving the water, it wasn't uncommon to find a small leech or two down near my toes. The bite itself was painless, and they are easily removed.

TREATMENT FOR LEECHES

Care needs to be taken when removing a leech. Similar to a tick, if removed improperly, the mouth area can actually be left in the bite itself. It is best to use your fingernail to gently pry the sucker away from the skin. While pulling them out manually is usually successful, other methods I found while researching this topic included pouring salt on them and applying a hot match to them. I've never tried either method, so feel free to experiment with them, but be warned that when they are violently disturbed, they will often regurgitate their stomach contents back into the wound when detaching. This virtually guarantees that the bite location will become infected. When the leech is (properly) removed, clean the site with soap and water to prevent any infection, as sometimes the bite location will bleed a little. In very rare occasions, the bite may become infected or an ulcer may develop. In these cases, medical attention should be sought. Fortunately, only a handful of cases of leeches transmitting pathogens to humans have been reported.

CHIGGERS

These annoying little creatures are in the same family as mites. They are microscopic and can be very troublesome. While the common vernacular refers to them as chiggers, they are also known as harvest mites, harvest bugs, harvest lice, mower's mites and red bugs. They are in the same arachnid 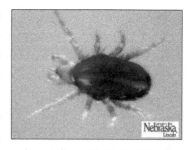 family as spiders and ticks. They are found from the southeastern United States to the midwest and love to hang around moist, grassy areas such as pastures, fields, forests, and even your yard. The babies are actually ones that bite. They are usually red, but can be orange or yellow as well. They are a whopping 0.3 millimeters long. They tend to stay in groups in grassy areas and attach themselves to prey as it passes by.

They tend to be most active during the warmer months, and die off when the temperature drops below 40 degrees. Once they have hitched a ride on your clothing they seek out the nearest patch of skin and go to town. Using sharp claws, they make tiny holes in the skin. They then inject a saliva that dissolves the skin cells. The resulting "mush" is food for them, and they will remain present for several days while eating. While they can bite anywhere on the body, the most common locations are in the form of clusters around the waist and lower legs. The initial bite(s) may be painless,

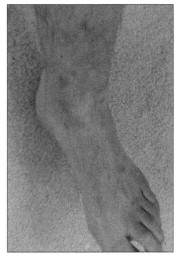

but within a few hours, the itch arrives in force. The itch can last for up to a week and will turn the skin red with bumps and blisters (as seen in the photo on the above right), and sometimes a rash that can take several weeks to heal. While they are not known to spread disease, the itching can lead to scratching that breaks the skin and can lead to infection.

TREATMENT FOR CHIGGERS

If you've been in an area that has chiggers and suspect you may have picked up some, it's best to do a full body check. If they are present, you will see tiny red dots moving around on your skin. The first step is to take a shower and scrub yourself clean with soap and water. Any clothes worn should be washed immediately. Treatment can be accomplished with anti-itch medications such as menthol, calamine lotion, and hydrocortisone creams. Antihistamine pills can also give relief as well. Most of the time, the problem clears up within a few days, but if itching and swelling continue or get worse, a steroid shot may be required, along with antibiotics if the bite location has become infected.

Chiggers can be avoided by taking similar precautions to prevent tick bites. Tucking in pant legs and wearing long sleeves can help prevent them latching on. Insect repellents such as DEET or permethrin can help ward them off as well. If you prefer natural deterrents, sprays made with essential oils such as citronella, tea tree, jojoba, geranium, or lemon grass have been proven to be effective.

CHAPTER FOUR

CRITTERS THAT WALK, STALK AND SLITHER

It should be obvious by now that there are tons of insects and other tiny creeping things that we may occasionally come into contact with while enjoying the great outdoors. This chapter deals with other animals that we may come into contact with that can potentially pose a threat to humans. We start with a discussion of the larger apex predators and move on to various snakes that are commonly encountered. In these types of situations, the best course forward is to keep the person calm and survey the situation. If it is safe to do so, move the victim out of the area and to a hospital or first responder as soon as possible. We will cover some first aid and trauma basics in another chapter that can be used to minimize the impact of an attack. When it comes to larger animal encounters, most attacks can be prevented by a healthy dose of situational awareness. If you encounter a bear or hog with babies, stay clear of them and do not come in between the mother and her young. If you are hiking in dangerous predator country, have some sort of deterrent on you at all times. Bear mace, bells, and air horns are relatively cheap and provide a decent level of protection.

If you are proficient with a firearm and it is legal in your area to carry, that is also another option to consider. Most predators will err on the side of caution when interacting with a human, so being aware of your surroundings will greatly reduce the likelihood of a negative encounter.

Most attacks by larger predators are a result of either territorial issues or hunger. Territorial issues can range from the aforementioned mother with babies, or could be an overly zealous male who sees anything other than a female of their species as a threat. Hunger can be a main catalyst as well, with campsites being tempting treats for a hungry predator. Properly securing food and cooking away from your main campsite are ways to reduce the likelihood of an interaction with a curious and hungry animal.

LARGE PREDATOR ENCOUNTERS

MOUNTAIN LIONS

While they were nearly hunted into extinction in some areas of the country, mountain lions are beginning to make a comeback. Typical habitat is in mountainous regions west of the Mississippi River, although many sightings have been reported in the southeast and northeast as well. Wildlife officials in my home state of Georgia have only recently acknowledged the possibility of cougars making their way back into the state, although there have been numerous sightings in my county alone. I was fortunate enough to catch a glimpse of one late one night as it was dragging a fresh roadkill deer carcass off into the woods, and weeks later the local high school experienced a scare as one was seen crossing across the practice field that borders a large ridge.

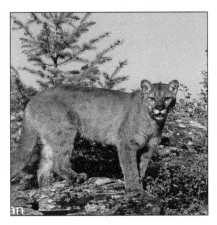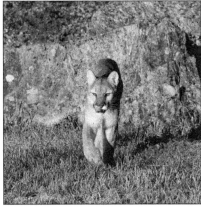

Also referred to as cougars, pumas, jaguars, and panthers, these animals are quite adept at stalking prey. They are typically ambush predators, preferring to stalk and attack from behind. Coloration on these big cats is typically various shades of brown and white, although darker varieties can be found among the various subspecies. Weight ranges from 100 pounds for the average grown female to 125 pounds for the males. The characteristic that sticks out the most about them is their long tails.

There have been around 125 confirmed cougar attacks in North America in the last 100 years, with around 30 of those being fatal. The best defense against cougar attacks is situational awareness. Cougars do not specifically target humans, as they have a natural aversion to us. However, it's obvious that encounters do happen, and there are several steps one can take to avoid a deadly encounter. Hiking in groups, keeping children in sight at all times, avoiding any fresh animal kills, and keeping dogs on leashes are good ways to stay out of a cougar's sights. Also, know the various signs of a cougar's presence, such as tracks, claw marks, and droppings. Most parks with cougar populations will have warnings with pictures at ranger stations and major trail heads.

PREVENTING AN ATTACK

If you do come face to face with one, waving your arms and trying to appear as large as possible while yelling loudly, maintaining eye contact and baring your teeth are ways to convince a curious cat that you are not the best of prey and they will typically move on. Do your best to provide the animal an avenue of escape so that it doesn't feel cornered. Since cougars prefer to ambush their prey, trusting that sixth sense that tells you that you are being watched can be invaluable. In the unlikely event that a cougar attacks you or someone in your party, fight back ferociously, aiming for the eyes and the face. Keep the neck covered if possible, as that's often the target of their attacks. After the attack is over, check the victim for injuries and apply first aid as necessary, keeping the victim as calm as possible and covered in order to prevent them from going into shock. The biggest concerns will be deep lacerations and bites from the cat's large claws and teeth. Stop the bleeding and clean the wound as well as possible, then cover it and wrap it with sterile pads and gauze or medical tape and seek more advanced medical care immediately.

BROWN / GRIZZLY BEARS

When it comes to bears in the continental United States, the Grizzly Bear reigns supreme. Depicted as a savage hunter and killer in many movies, it definitely can cause a person to panic if they encounter one. Before we go any farther, it should be pointed out that the Brown Bear and Grizzly Bear are technically the same species. The only differences are their size and the habitat they reside in. Brown Bears are typically found in the coastal regions whereas Grizzly Bears are found much more inland. When it comes to size, the Brown Bear can weigh in at over

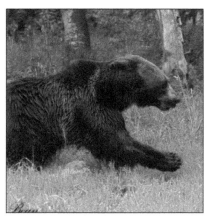 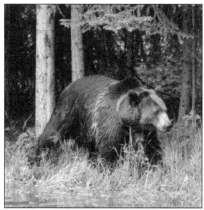

1,000 pounds, whereas the Grizzly is rarely seen over 900 pounds. Females usually weigh about ⅓ less than their male counterparts. As far as coloration, various shades of brown can be found on these bears, mostly dependent on their region.

BROWN / GRIZZLY BEAR ATTACKS AND PREVENTION

When it comes to human and Brown Bear encounters, most of the time the bear will bluff by growling or snapping it's teeth and may run at the human but turning away at the last moment. Over the past several decades, there have been between 1 and 3 attacks annually. Most encounters result in a stalemate, with both bear and human going their separate ways. In the event where an actual physical attack took place, the result was almost always a fatality. The most aggressive attacks tend to be when a human accidentally gets near a mother with cubs. If you do happen upon bear cubs in the wild, immediately leave the area. Do not run, as it could trigger a chase response, but exit as soon as you can. Wherever cubs are present, the mother is sure to be close at hand.

If you do find yourself staring down an angry or aggressive Brown Bear, there are steps you can take to de-escalate the situation. One measure is to stand still and slowly wave your arms up and down and speak in a slow but firm way to help the bear realize you are not prey. Never scream or try to imitate the sound the bear is making, as this can trigger an aggressive response. Do not climb a tree, as Brown Bears and Grizzlies are expert climbers. As with cougars, make yourself appear as large as possible by moving to higher ground. If the bear remains stationary, begin exiting the area by walking away slowly and sideways, to allow you to keep an eye on the bear. If it starts to follow or bluff, stand your ground once more. Given an opportunity to escape, most bears will choose to end the encounter by walking away.

However, if the bear decides to attack, there are a few things you can do to protect yourself. Bear spray should always accompany any hiker in bear territory. If the bear charges or attacks, deploy the spray into the bear's face and eyes. In most cases, this is enough to end the attack. If the bear does attack, do not drop your backpack, as this will serve to protect you from the force of the bear's impact. Brown Bears prefers to attack from behind and typically go for the neck and head. Put your hands around your neck and lie flat on the ground and play dead. Extend your legs out in order to prevent the bear from turning you over. Most attacks will end by this point. If, and only if, the attack persists, fight back with everything you have in you, as it has truly gotten to the point of a life or death situation.

Remain still until the bear discontinues the attack and leaves the area. Immediately assess the damage to yourself or any member of your party that was attacked and begin first aid treatment. Identify and stop any excessive bleeding, utilizing a tourniquet if present, and keep the victim as calm and still as possible. Utilize a blanket or other clothing to keep the victim warm and from going into shock. Clean and cover the wounds as best as you can. Call in advanced medical support if you are in an area accessible by vehicle or helicopter, or slowly and methodically move the victim to a place where emergency medical personnel can meet you and take over. If hiking or camping alone in Brown Bear country, ensure that a tourniquet is part of your first aid gear and is of a type that can be applied easily with one hand. If you find yourself bleeding profusely after a bear attack, a tourniquet will likely be the deciding factor between living and dying. Far too many people overlook the importance of adequate medical gear when venturing into apex predator territory. People will spend hundreds or thousands of dollars and hours of research on the most high tech camping gear, clothing, and footwear. While there is nothing wrong with this, please ensure that you give the same amount of research and scrutiny to the type of first aid gear that you will be carrying in the backcountry.

It should be noted that many outdoorsmen and outdoorswomen carry a firearm of some sort while in bear country. While this can be an effective way of stopping an attack, the shooter needs to be proficient with his weapon. No exceptions. Too many people tend to buy a firearm and fire it once or twice and then feel that they are invincible. Trying to hit an area the size of a bear's head or heart is difficult enough under hunting conditions, but in a life or death struggle, may only make things worse by wounding an already enraged bear. If you do carry a firearm, ensure that it is in a suitable caliber and that it is carried in a manner that allows quick access should an attack occur. Having a .44 Magnum revolver in the bottom of your backpack will do you no good if you find yourself being mauled by an angry bear. Also, if you carry a firearm, you should still carry bear spray as a first line of defense. In many states and parks, shooting a bear without being able to prove your life was in danger can result in heavy fines and penalties. Always have a less than lethal option at hand. In addition, firearm laws vary from state to state, so if you decide to carry one, always ensure that you are in accordance with state and federal law.

BLACK BEARS

Found throughout the entire continent of North America, the Black Bear is the smallest of the bears found in the United States. With males averaging 150 to 300 pounds on average, they are definitely dwarfed by some of their bigger cousins out west. As their name implies, most are black in color, although color patterns ranging from solid white to cinnamon have been observed. Their preferred habitat is forested regions, which is one reason that there are far more black bear and human

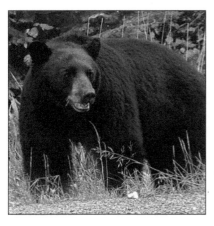
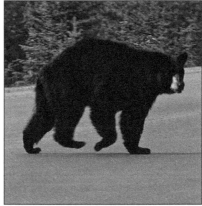

interactions than with other species of North American bears. Another reason is that they vastly outnumber the other bear species, leading to larger populations sharing the woods with hikers, fishermen, and campers.

BLACK BEAR ATTACKS AND PREVENTION

Most Black Bear encounters end with the bear huffing and bluff charging and then ambling back off into the woods. With their populations larger than other bears, they are more exposed to humans, often exploring human settlements in search of food. Most attacks are a direct result of a Black Bear seeking out food, such as in a campsite or out of a garbage can at the back of a house. Since bears of this type learn to associate humans with the availability of food, encounters are more numerous. If you have spent any time in national parks where Black Bears are present, you will likely see all manner of signs and measures warning campers and hikers to keep garbage cans closed and secured and food out of the reach of bears.

When traveling through Black Bear habitat, ensure that you take the proper precautions. Staying on the trail, carrying bear spray, and traveling in groups are good ways to keep a curious bear from investigating any further. However, in the event that a Black Bear does attack, many of the same rules apply to surviving an attack from a Brown Bear. For instance, making oneself appear larger and more threatening will often discourage a further attack. Making noise such as yelling or using an air horn will also serve to discourage an attack. Keep direct eye contact with the bear and do not run, as doing so could trigger an aggressive response. If the bear continues to approach, deploying bear spray is the next move. If the Black Bear initiates a physical attack, the rules differ from a Brown Bear encounter. With a Black Bear, the victim should fight back using any means necessary, concentrating on the eyes and face. Black Bears often rise up on two legs and seek to knock their victims down, following up with bites to the arms or legs and, finally, a strike to the head to finish them off. Playing dead in these scenarios will only intensify the number and extent of any injuries inflicted. There have been only 25 fatal Black Bear attacks over the last 20 years, so fighting back may very well make the most difference in your chances of survival.

Once the attack has ceased, and the animal is gone from the area, immediately examine yourself or any other victim for obvious injuries. Any excessive bleeding will need to be dealt with first, followed up by examination for any broken bones.

Apply a tourniquet to halt excessive bleeding and a splint to any broken bones in order to keep them immobilized. The victim should be kept calm and covered to prevent shock while advanced medical help is sought. If possible, carry the victim to a location where EMS personnel can meet you and administer further care.

WOLVES

The most commonly-encountered wolf species in North America is the Grey Wolf, also referred to as the Timber Wolf. Their historic range is west of the Mississippi River from Texas to Canada. Their coloration can range from nearly solid white to almost black, with most animals in a greyish black color scheme. The males are the largest of the species, weighing in at up to 180 pounds when fully grown. Females are quite a bit smaller, coming in at 120 pounds when fully grown. Their howl is what stands out about them to most people who venture into wolf country, as it can truly be a spine-tingling sensation when first encountering it.

Fortunately, wolf attacks on humans are relatively rare. The last recorded fatality in North America was in 2010. However, attacks do occur from time to time, and tend to be more from a predatory response to a human entering their territory. The attack may stem simply from a human being present, or the attack may be driven by hunger. Wolves have been observed stalking hikers and campers in remote locations, often focusing their efforts on lone hikers or small groups.

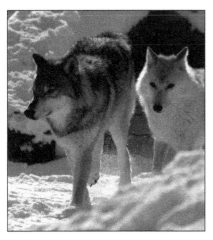 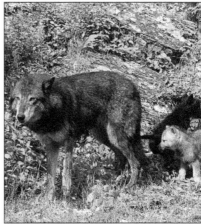

WOLF ATTACKS AND PREVENTION

Since many wolf attacks stem from hunger, cooking and disposing of food scraps away from your primary camp site is imperative. Also, properly storing food where it is not accessible to wolves is a rule always to be followed. If you hear a lone wolf howl, never respond, as the animal may mistake you for another in it's pack and come running towards the sound. Since wolves hunt in packs, they often howl to each other as a form of communication, helping them to track prey. Drawing attention to yourself is the last thing you want to do in a situation like this. If you are hiking through wolf country and come upon an animal kill, leave the area as soon as possible, as a wolf, bear, or other large predator is likely in the area.

If you find yourself face to face with a single wolf or a pack, there are some measures you can take to de-escalate the situation. First, if the wolf has not noticed you, slowly and quietly back away and leave the area. If the wolf has noticed you, appear as large as possible by waving your arms and yelling, while throwing rocks or any other objects you can find nearby. Avoid making eye contact with the wolf, as they will see this as a challenge of dominance. They will often give signs as to an impending attack, such as snarling, growling, and the bristling of the hair on their back. If you are able, climb onto a rock or up a tree, as wolves are not climbers. However, they are patient hunters, and may hang around for some time before losing interest and moving on.

If you find yourself under attack, utilize any weapon possible while protecting your face and neck. If you are carrying a firearm, firing off a shot may very well end the attack as the noise will scare off the wolf. If not, it will be necessary to shoot to kill. Knives, rocks, branches, and anything else that can be used for a weapon should be utilized. Their most sensitive areas are the nose and eyes. Some survival experts recommend jamming your arm into their mouth as a last ditch effort to stop an attack, under the theory that the wolf will not be able to bite or breathe and will break off the attack. In a truly nightmare scenario where you find yourself under attack by multiple wolves, it's imperative to take out the alpha, which is usually the largest and strongest animal, or else the rest of the pack will continue to attack. Wolves are cunning and determined predators, and while the chances of an attack are extremely low, it's important to know what you are up against when entering their territory.

When it comes to first aid following an attack, the formula for other large predators still rings true. Ensure that any excessive bleeding is controlled and stopped, any lacerations are cleaned and bandaged, and the victim is evacuated from the area in the quickest manner possible.

WILD BOAR

Wild Boar are not a species that is native to North America. Brought over by European settlers, many eventually escaped and turned feral. It's estimated that there are approximately 5 million wild boar in the continental United States. In many states, they are considered a nuisance and the hunting of them is encouraged due to the property damage they cause. In addition, they can carry upwards of 20 different diseases that can be transferred to humans that eat undercooked meat. They also carry parasites and diseases that can easily spread to domesticated pigs and other livestock animals.

These diseases include the following:

• Pseudorabies Virus (PRV)
• Swine brucellosis (Brucella suis)
• Bovine tuberculosis (TB)
• FADs
• African swine fever
• Classical swine fever (Hog Cholera)
• Foot and Mouth Disease

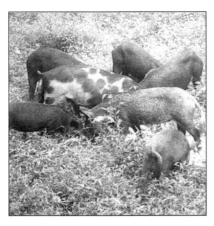
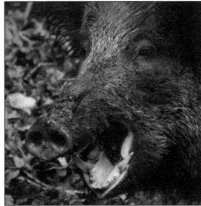

Size ranges from 170 to 220 pounds for males and slightly smaller for females, although there have been several killed by hunters that were much larger, some up to 1,000 pounds. Both male and female boar have tusks, with the males having much larger, curved tusks. Their range in the continental United States is virtually all of the southern half of the country. However, due to their invasive nature, their habitat is constantly expanding. Their coloration can range from solid blacks and browns, to various color combinations of black, brown, white, gray, and pink.

As with the other large predators that we have discussed, the likelihood of an attack by a wild boar is relatively small. There have only been four confirmed fatalities from a wild boar attack in the United States since the late 1800's, and most of them have been from a wounded boar attacking a hunter. However, non-fatal attacks do occur, and the majority of them have been in recent decades as the population increases and they are more likely to come into contact with people. The typical triggers apply to wild boar with males attacking due to being surprised or cornered and females attacking when they feel that their young are in danger.

WILD BOAR ATTACKS AND PREVENTION

Most confrontations with wild boar end with the person simply backing away and diffusing the situation. Never approach one or try to feed it. If you encounter piglets, leave them alone, as the mother is nearby and will likely turn aggressive due to seeing you as a threat. While most attacks are from a single animal, there have been documented cases of multiple boar attacking at once.

If you encounter a wild boar and it begins to approach you, stand as tall as possible and shout at it. This will more than likely break off the confrontation. If the boar is insistent and begins to charge, the best course of action is to climb a rock or the nearest tree. Boar can charge at over 10 miles per hour, so if you don't have a chance to find higher ground, try your best to sidestep the animal to avoid the tusks. Male boars typically target the thigh with their tusks, inflicting as many painful stabs and cuts as possible. Female boars typically will growl and her shoulders and tail will stand up erect. Since their tusks are smaller, they tend to bite their victims. With either sex, the attack will be brutal and quick, as they tend to break off and evaluate their victim. It's important to try to remain upright if possible, as they will try to knock a human off their feet in order to obtain the advantage over them and inflict as much damage as possible. In this scenario, fight back with whatever means possible. More often than not, the mauling will end when the boar decides further aggression is not justified. Most attacks are over in less than one minute.

When it comes to first aid, there are a number of scenarios to consider. If there are multiple puncture wounds, it is imperative to stop the bleeding as soon as possible, while checking to insure that no major arteries have been affected. Since the tusks can cut and slash, they can do just as much damage as a knife blade. Keep the victim as calm as possible, and immediately get them medical attention, even if the wounds seem minor. Any contact with wild boar saliva can carry with it the risk of a transmittable disease such as:

• Leptospirosis
• Brucellosis
• E. coli
• Salmonellosis
• Toxoplasmosis
• Rabies (which is discussed in the next section)
• Swine Influenza viruses
• Trichinosis
• Giardiasis
• Cryptosporidiosis

Victims of any wild boar attack should be taken to a medical facility where they can be tested to ensure that they have not contracted a disease due to their encounter.

OTHER ANIMALS

When it comes to other animals, the likelihood of a dangerous encounter is rather slim. Here in the south, there are occasional coyote attacks, usually on small children. These are very isolated occurrences, as normally they seize on the opportunity when their prey is separated from a group. Most animals will avoid humans when we come across them in their environment. However, there is a condition that leads to negative human / animal encounters and that is when an animal is suffering from rabies.

Rabies is a disease that attacks the central nervous system and ultimately winds up in the brain. The early symptoms of the disease in humans is similar to that of the flu, including fever, weakness, and general discomfort. As the disease progresses, more serious symptoms appear and include insomnia, anxiety, confusion, partial paralysis, excitation, hallucinations, agitation, hypersalivation, difficulty swallowing, and hydrophobia (a fear of water). Once these symptoms have begun, death usually occurs within a matter of days. If rabies is a concern in an area, most parks will have info and pictures of the animals to be cautious around.

The animals most likely to be carriers of the disease are as follows:

RACCOONS

The racoon is one of North America's most adaptable animals. Found all over the country, these critters can make a home in the forest or the city. They are natural climbers and are typically most active at night. They are notorious for stealing food from outside cats, dogs, and smaller livestock animals. Weight typically ranges from 10 to 30 pounds, although there have been specimens observed as large as 60 pounds.

They are most easily recognized by their distinctive black "mask" across their eyes as well as their banded tail. Their bodies are most often colored a mix of black, brown and white, although there have been solid white and brown specimens observed in the wild as well. Their disposition can range from curious to aggres-

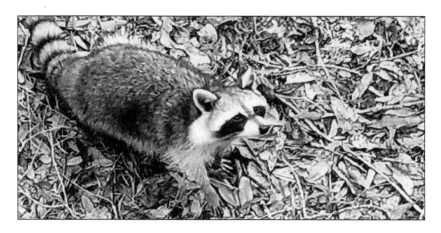

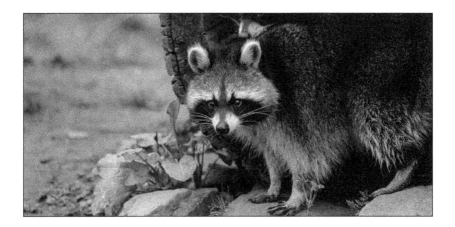

sive, so leaving them alone is the best course of action. They will typically growl and hiss to deter any further intrusion, with biting as a last resort. In addition to rabies, raccoons can also transmit the following diseases to humans and domestic animals:

• Raccoon Roundworm
• Leptospirosis
• Canine Distemper

SKUNKS

Found throughout the United States and Canada, the skunk is certainly an animal that most everyone can recognize. With their distinctive stripe, they are easily identifiable. Coloration can range from black to brown with their white stripe, although albino skunks are not uncommon. Typical size is 6 to 10 pounds. They prefer to make their homes in places they can burrow, such as downed trees, areas with heavy vegetation, and will even make a burrow in the ground if no cover is deemed suitable. They typically find an area within close proximity to a water source and will remain within a two mile range of that area.

They are mostly nocturnal, which helps to limit their interaction with humans. While most people associate them with their ability to spray a foul, long-lasting odor, they actually save that as a last line of defense. If they are disturbed or are caught out with their young, they will typically growl, spit, stomp the ground, and

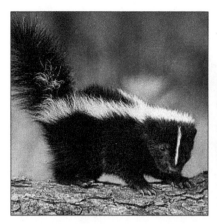
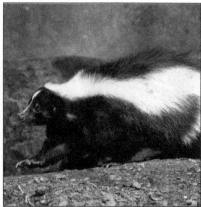

shake their fur as a deterrence. Only when they feel no other option is available will they turn around, lift their tail, and spray. They can spray up to 10 feet and the odor is detectable for up to a mile and a half. While they are known carriers of rabies, the bite of a skunk can have other risks to humans and pets such as:

- Leptospirosis
- Canine Distemper
- Canine Hepatitis
- Intestinal Roundworm

BATS

With more than 40 distinct species present, bats are found throughout all regions and habitats of North America. They can be just as prevalent in rural areas as they can larger cities. Size ranges from a few ounces to a pound, with wingspans of up

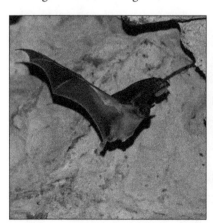
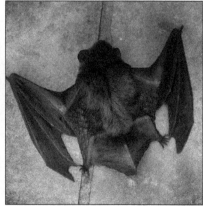

to 13 inches in some species. They are a nocturnal mammal, spending most of their time in dark areas such as caves or abandoned structures. They use a form of radar called echolocation to seek out insects to eat. Coloration is typically brown and black, or a mixture of the two. While healthy bats will not attack a human, their feces poses a risk. Numerous diseases such as salmonella and leptospirosis can be transmitted through contact with bat fecal matter, so if you happen upon an area where bats are active, it's best to limit any exposure, as even the dust from dried feces can contaminate the surrounding air.

COYOTES

The coyote is another animal that has learned to thrive in both rural and urban environments. Resembling a medium sized dog, the coyote is typically colored in a black or greyish-brown color scheme. They range in size from 25 to 40 pounds and can run up to 40 miles an hour for short bursts. They are adaptable to both woodland and open environments and have begun to be found in major urban environments. They are opportunistic predators, often eating rabbits, squirrels and other woodland creatures, in addition to chickens, small livestock, and even household pets. They often travel in packs and use howling, barking, and yelping as various forms of communication.

Encounters with humans are rare with healthy coyotes, but they do happen occasionally. Normally their extraordinary senses of hearing and smell alert them well in advance that people are present. Most attacks on humans are due to the

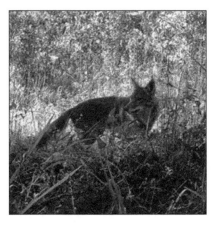
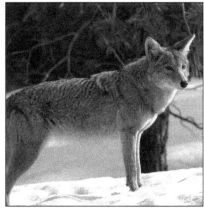

presence of the rabies virus in an animal. In addition to rabies, coyotes are also known to be carriers of:

- Tularemia
- Canine Distemper
- Canine Hepatitis
- Mange
- A wide variety of parasites

Since coyotes often target household animals, it's imperative that pet owners vaccinate their animals against rabies and if an encounter occurs, they take the pet to a veterinarian as soon as possible.

FOXES

There are four types of foxes present in North America: The Grey Fox, Red Fox, Arctic Fox, and Kit Fox.The Red Fox is the most prevalent and most frequently encountered. Typical weight is 20 to 30 pounds, with the other types weighing less, all the way down to an average of 5 pounds for the Kit Fox. Their color schemes virtually match their names, with the Arctic Fox being solid white and the Kit Fox is found with a reddish-brown or a greyish-brown scheme. They typically eat small rodents and some plants and fruits. They are one of the most intelligent canines on earth. Their habitat is as varied as the different types, yet they are very adaptable to areas near humans. Some have even been observed stalking farmers as they mow their fields, knowing that small rodents and rabbits will be disturbed and flee the

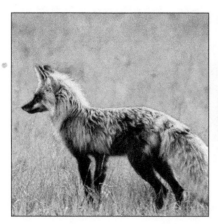
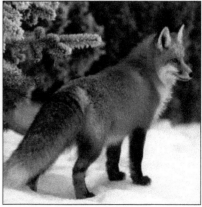

noise. They are opportunistic as well, going after chickens and other birds typically found on farms. They often hunt alone and are primarily nocturnal.

Healthy foxes pose no threat to humans, although they will attack household pets if the opportunity arises. While known for being a carrier of rabies, foxes also carry other diseases such as:

• Tularemia
• Roundworm
• Tapeworm
• Toxocariasis
• Mange

As with coyotes, healthy foxes rarely interact with humans, as their superior senses of hearing and smell allow them to be long gone before an interaction occurs. Only when rabid do attacks occur.

INTERACTIONS WITH RABID ANIMALS

Last summer, a hiker on a trail in middle Georgia encountered a coyote that was acting particularly aggressive. Daytime encounters are not common, and usually result in the coyote running away, so this immediately concerned the hiker. It attacked him and he had to dispatch it with his pocket knife. The coyote was sent off to be tested for rabies, and the hiker was immediately treated as a precaution. He recovered fully and the coyote tested positive for rabies.

When outdoors, if you happen upon an animal that is acting unusual, it's best to leave it alone and report it to your local fish and game agency. Never try to trap or catch the animal, as you will likely be bitten or scratched in the process. Animals suffering from the disease will exhibit a myriad of unusual behavior, such as extreme aggression or extreme calmness, sometimes approaching a human as if to seek attention. Sometimes they have the stereotypical foaming at the mouth and may have trouble walking or standing upright. If you are an unfortunate victim of one of these strange-acting animals, there are steps that you can take to ensure that you are safe from the disease. First, immediately clean the bite area to remove any additional saliva that may be present. Second, seek professional medical help immediately so that the rabies vaccination regimen can be started. The success rate is extremely high, provided that the victim not delay the initiation of treatment.

CRITTERS THAT SLITHER

We will now take a look at the various types of venomous snakes that one might encounter in the wilderness. Where we have had thousands of species of insects to deal with, there are only four main species of venomous snakes in North America: rattlesnakes, copperheads, cottonmouths, and coral snakes. While there are between 7,000 and 8,000 people bitten annually in the United States, there are only around 5 fatalities. Most often, snakes in general will avoid humans and will only bite when they feel cornered and threatened. While they will often make an impressive display utilizing hissing, rattling, puffing up, and other theatrics, if left alone, they will rarely pursue a human and both of you can go about your business.

RATTLESNAKES

There are 32 separate species of rattlesnakes in North America. From the massive eastern diamondback rattlesnake to the diminutive pygmy rattler, there are many species to be aware of. Since there are such a variety of sizes and color patterns among the different species, we encourage researching which species live in your area. This will allow you to more readily identify what type of rattlesnakes you may potentially encounter. The official Audubon Society field guide is very good (https://www.audubon.org/national-audubon-society-field-guides). They have comprehensive field guides for pretty much any animal, aquatic, or insect species on earth. They feature color photos and habitat information. I still have the one that my father gave me as a boy, since I was enthralled with snakes and caught any I could get my hands on.

Most all of them prefer areas of cover, such as rocky terrain where they can nest in groups during the colder seasons. They can also be encountered in areas with thick ground cover and densely forested regions. Some species even prefer sandy, coastal regions. They are known for their namesake rattles on their tails, which they use as a warning to deter predators. The older the snake, the more rattles will be present. The most commonly-encountered rattlesnakes are as follows:

DIAMONDBACK

The Diamondback Rattlesnake is easily identified by its distinctive diamond pattern on their backs. There are both Eastern and Western species, with the Eastern having a sharper, more clear pattern with distinct brown, black, and even yellowish coloration. The Western Diamondback still retains the distinctive pattern, but is often more of a subdued coloration with layers of brown. Size is typically in the 4-5 feet range in adults, but are often found up to 8 feet in length. The Eastern Diamondback is found mainly in the southeast, whereas the Western Diamondback is found mostly west of the Mississippi River.

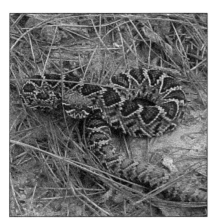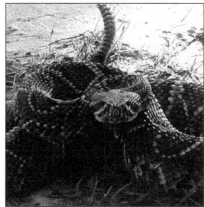

Diamondback rattlesnakes typically shy away from humans, only biting when taunted or cornered. They will often coil up and rattle to bluff their prey into leaving them alone. They can strike up to one third of their overall body length, so giving them a wide berth is the best way to avoid a bite. The Eastern Diamondback has the distinction of causing the most snakebite deaths in the United States. Not surprisingly, the Western Diamondback is a very close second place.

TIMBER (ALSO REFERRED TO AS A CANEBRAKE)

Timber Rattlesnakes are mostly found in the southeastern United States, but can be found in some midwestern states. For whatever reason, their habitat excludes the state of Florida. The Canebrake Rattlesnake is the same species but has a slightly different coloration and is found in the sandy coastal plains of the southeastern United States. The Timber Rattlesnake is mostly brown with black chevron bands and a black tail. The Canebrake Rattlesnake is mostly grey in color with the same black chevrons and black tail. The Canebrake is also known to have a distinctive brown, yellow, orange, and even pink line going down the center of it's back. The size for adults of both is around 4-5 feet with the largest coming in at a little over 6 feet.

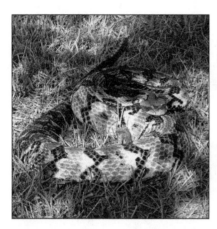 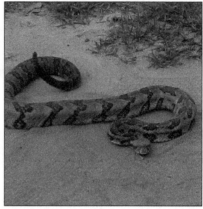

Similar to Diamondback Rattlesnakes, Timber and Canebrake Rattlesnakes will avoid humans if at all possible. When confronted or disturbed, they will coil and rattle in an effort to scare off a person, even more theatrically than the Diamondback. Only when directly threatened or if a person wanders right up on one will they bite.

PYGMY

The Pygmy Rattlesnake is the smallest of the rattlesnakes that we will discuss. With an average length of 15 to 24 inches, this one is easy to miss. There are eastern and western versions of the snake, which give them a fairly wide range in the southern half of the United States. Coloration is typically a greyish background with alternating black and reddish-orange spots across the back and sides. They are found in a variety of habitats, ranging from pine forests to sandy coastal regions. They prefer regions where water is nearby and will often take over the burrows of native turtles.

While the Pygmy Rattlesnake does have a rattle on its tail, it is not often heard. In fact, the snake prefers to remain silent and still when potential prey is close. If it continues to feel threatened, it will often move it's head from side to side in an effort to bluff the predator. With fangs that are small in comparison to other spe-

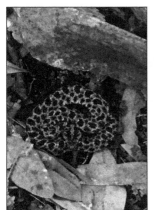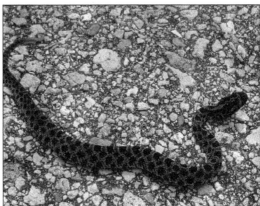

cies of rattlesnakes, the Pygmy Rattlesnake does not typically deliver a fatal bite if provoked. That being said, a bite from one of these diminutive snakes is still one of the most unpleasant experiences that you could possibly have, so if you happen upon one, be sure to leave it alone and both of you can go about your business.

PRAIRIE

Sometimes referred to as the Great Plains Rattlesnake, The Prairie Rattlesnake occupies a habitat in the middle of North America, from southwestern Canada all the way down into northern Mexico. Typical size for an adult is around 3 feet, with the largest recorded around 5 feet. As their name implies, they mostly prefer grasslands and prairies, but will also make a home in forested areas, rocky terrain, and alongside streams. Their coloration ranges from a yellowish-brown to an olive green body with brown or black blotches that flatten out into rings near the tail, with males typically having more rings than females.

Since they tend to be smaller than some of the other members of the rattlesnake family, their venom glands are smaller. However, when they do bite they tend to inject up to 50% of the available venom, which is more than enough to cause a fatality if medical help is delayed or unavailable. As with other rattlesnakes, they

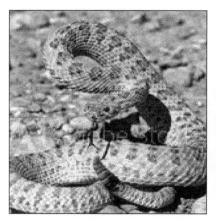 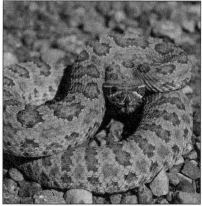

are not naturally aggressive towards humans. Only when startled or threatened will they strike. Their typical defense posture is to coil and rattle in an attempt to dissuade their attacker from further aggression.

SIDEWINDER

Sometimes referred to as the Horned Rattlesnake, the Sidewinder Rattlesnake is typically found in the southwestern region of the United States and into northern Mexico. Typical length is around 2 feet. They possess the unique ability to change their coloration to match their surroundings through a process known as meta-chrosis. As a result, they can appear yellowish-brown, greyish, and even pinkish bodies with rhombus shaped blotches along their back and sides. As their name-sake implies, they are known for their ability to crawl sideways across the terrain, leaving a J-shaped impression. They prefer a habitat with wide open terrain and sand or loose soil in order to enable their sidewinding locomotion.

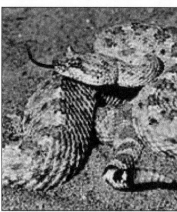 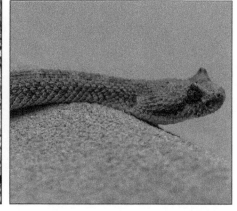

While capable of delivering bites that are fatal, this rattlesnake is similar to all it's other relatives in that it will not provoke an attack. Only when threatened or picked up will it strike. As with all other species of rattlesnakes, it will often rattle to intimidate any predator in the hopes of driving it away. If you happen upon one of these interesting snakes, simply leaving it alone is your best option.

PREVENTION AND TREATMENT FOR RATTLESNAKE BITES

As mentioned previously, when threatened, the rattlesnake will coil up and rattle its tail in order to frighten off predators. However, it's not guaranteed that the snake will rattle if threatened. Sometimes they remain perfectly still in the hopes that the predator will move on. Case in point is this very healthy female timber rattlesnake that I almost sat on in a vacant cabin along a local hiking trail. I never noticed it, and it never rattled, even though I almost sat on the small bench it was curled up under. Needless to say, it was a bit of a shock when my son yelled "Dad, there's a snake!!" We all got out of the cabin safely and then I went back for pictures, much to my wife's dismay (I took a stick in with me to try and get it to stretch out, but was overruled by my better half).

If you encounter a rattlesnake and are bitten, there are several steps that you can take to minimize the trauma. While about 25% of venomous snake bites are "dry bites" where no venom is injected, it's best to treat every bite from a venomous snake as a serious condition and seek medical treatment. A bite from a juvenile is actually the most dangerous, as they have not 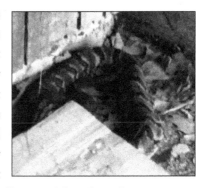 developed the ability to control their venom flow yet. After a bite, the victim may experience symptoms such as swelling and bruising at the bite site, numbness in the face and limbs, weakness, nausea and vomiting, sweating, excessive salivating, lightheadedness, blurred vision and difficulty breathing.

When it comes to first aid for a rattlesnake bite, there are a lot of dangerous myths that have floated around for years. For instance, those snake bite kits that you find in the camping section at big box stores are useless and may actually do more harm than good. In addition, cutting the bite site and attempting to suck the venom out is an equally bad idea, as is applying a tourniquet. The proper first aid procedures are to stay calm and try to get away from the snake as soon as possible. If it is safe to do so, try to get a good look at the snake so that the first responders can have as much info as possible regarding what type of venomous snake has bitten you. If you are in a group, keep the victim stable and calm, but don't elevate the bite location above heart level, as this can spread the venom to the heart quicker. If you are alone and bitten, it is imperative that you remain as calm as possible and collect your nerves before slowly beginning to leave the area to seek medical help. If possible, draw a circle around the bite location and write down the time you were bitten. This will allow first responders and medical personnel to monitor the progression of the swelling at the bite site. Remove any restrictive clothing near the bite location and clean it and lightly bandage it. Most bites result in full re-covery, even if antivenin is required. Most people who suffer complications are the ones who allow themselves to panic, thereby spreading the venom throughout the bloodstream much more quickly. It's recommended that a rattlesnake bite victim receive medical help within 30 minutes of being bitten.

COPPERHEAD

This snake has the dubious distinction of inflicting the most bites annually in the United States. This is due in large part to the fact that their distinctive shades of brown allow them to completely blend into their native surroundings. I've walked up on them before and not even noticed their presence until I was virtually on top of them. Adults range in size from 2-4 feet and have a stocky body. They are found throughout the United States, mostly in the eastern half. They are common in wooded environments, but can also be found near water. I've seen them swim across creeks and ponds many times. They are known to come up around homes, barns, gardens, and flower beds, where a lot of their interactions with humans occur.

Their primary defense mechanism is to sit perfectly still and blend into their en-vironment. My son was walking one of our dogs a few years ago and they walked up on a large one sitting at the base of a pine tree. It virtually disappeared into the background of pine needles and dirt. My son almost stepped on it before noticing

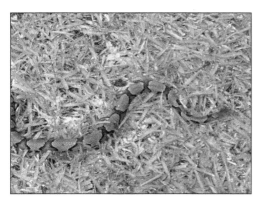 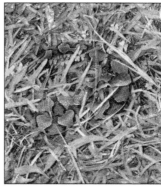

it. It stayed coiled, but didn't move as he slowly backed away. Most bites occur when the snake feels cornered and threatened. As a last ditch effort to frighten predators, a copperhead will vibrate its tail rapidly, sometimes causing it to be mistaken for a rattlesnake.

TREATMENT FOR COPPERHEAD BITES

The bite of a copperhead is rarely fatal in adults, yet the pain is intense and is often long-lasting. Other symptoms include tingling, throbbing, swelling, and severe nausea. Damage can occur to both muscle and bone tissue, especially if the bite occurs on an outer extremity such as feet and hands. I had a good friend in high school who was bitten in the finger as he reached to move some brush. He was in the hospital for a few days and said it felt like he had the worst version of the flu possible. First aid procedures are to immobilize the area and ensure that it stays lower than the heart. As with other venomous snakes, it's imperative that the victim remain calm, as this will slow the spread of the venom around your system. As discussed with rattlesnakes, never try to apply a tourniquet or suck the venom out. The bite area should be cleaned and bandaged and medical help sought immediately. While certainly an animal to avoid, the venom of the copperhead is known to possess certain cancer-fighting properties and may one day be used to treat certain types of the disease.

COTTONMOUTH

Also referred to as a water moccasin, these snakes are found in and around bodies of water. It's name comes from the fact that when they assume a defensive posture, they open their jaws wide to reveal the white insides of their mouth. They are masterful swimmers and can be found in color schemes from solid black or brown to various-colored bands that cause it to be commonly confused with many non-venomous water snakes. They can be told apart by the fact that the cottonmouth swims with the majority of its body above water, where the non-venomous water snakes will swim with only their head above water. They range in size from 2 to 4 feet in length and are usually quite stocky. They are native mainly to the southeast, where they can usually be found basking in the sun on logs or rocks at the edge of rivers and creeks.

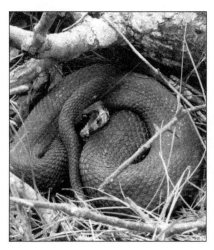 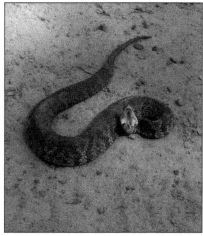

While most non-venomous water snakes will flee from predators, cottonmouths will typically stand their ground and spread their mouth open to deter a potential predator. Despite this aggressive posturing, they rarely bite unless stepped on or picked up. Just recently, there was a story in the local paper where a man was bitten by a cottonmouth while at a popular swimming hole. Thankfully, he was evacuated by ATV to the trailhead where an ambulance was able to take him to be treated at an area hospital. There was another story that made headlines a few years ago when a young man in Florida was bitten after he caught a cottonmouth and, for reasons unknown, attempted to kiss it. You can imagine what happened next. The result was a dangerously swollen face and a lengthy hospital stay and recovery. It should go without saying that this is why it's advisable to leave these snakes alone, up to and including public displays of affection. After all, they're really just not that into you.

TREATMENT FOR COTTONMOUTH BITES

A cottonmouth bite will typically show multiple symptoms in the victim. The limbs will begin swelling very soon after the bite is inflicted, which is followed by a painful itching sensation. Chills, increased heart rate and trembling soon follow. Finally, partial paralysis will occur in the part of the body affected by the bite. If you are unfortunate enough to sustain a bite from a cottonmouth, the following steps should be taken to ensure a successful recovery. As with all venomous snake bites, the number one first aid step is to keep the victim calm in order to slow the spread of venom to the other parts of the body. Clean the bite area and apply a bandage around it to keep any other debris out of the open wound. Remove any constricting clothing to ensure that the swelling is not any more painful than it has to be. Be mindful to monitor the bite area for any color changes or additional swelling. Medical treatment should be administered as soon as possible after the bite. The survivability of a cottonmouth bite is very high if medical treatment is obtained in a timely manner, although there are a handful of deaths every year as well. Some articles I've come across recommend that you try to catch and kill the snake that inflicted the bite in order to help hospital staff better determine what course of antivenin to administer. This, put quite mildly, is horrible advice. If you can make a positive id, (be that a visual id, cell phone photo, etc.) then relay that information to first responders. Chasing after the snake or trying to dispatch it under extreme stress will likely result in the need for two people being treated for snakebite instead of just one.

MISIDENTIFICATION

The cottonmouth is often confused with a number of similar-appearing water snakes, such as this Northern Water Snake. While the pupil of the eye is a good way to tell venomous snakes from non-venomous snakes, most people don't prefer to get that close. The shape of the head is not always indicative, either. Non-venomous water snakes will routinely flatten their head similar to that of a cottonmouth when they feel threatened, leading to many being killed simply 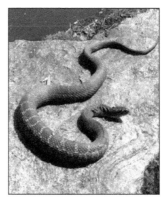 due to their appearance. Water snakes are notorious for being aggressive if messed with too much (I tried to pick this guy up twice and he simply wasn't having it), so it's best just to leave them to themselves and avoid a potential encounter, be it with a non-venomous or a venomous snake.

CORAL SNAKE

Last on our list of venomous snakes in North America is the diminutive Coral Snake. Their size is usually around 3 feet when fully grown, and their color scheme has alternating red, yellow, and black bands. You may have heard the saying "red and black, venom lack; red and yellow, kill a fellow" in regards to identifying them. This applies to the North American Coral Snake only, as some species in other countries have differing color schemes. It is often confused with the scarlet snake, the milk snake, and some species of kingsnakes, all of which are non-venomous. It's range is primarily the deep southeast, with separate Arizona and Texas species also found in the southwest.

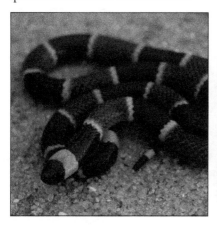 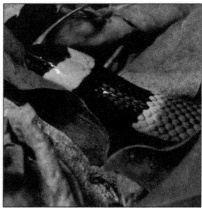

The Coral Snake prefers to remain elusive, often hiding in burrows or under cover on the forest floor. When it comes to their bite, they differ from the other three venomous species that we have discussed so far. Their fangs are rather small in comparison, and the Coral Snake relies on biting and making chewing motions while doing so in order to deliver their venom. Their elusiveness and lack of aggression are the reason that they account for less than one percent of snake bites in the United States each year. They prefer to flee when encountering a predator and only bite as a last result. However, there are still between 15 and 25 bites annually, and the results for those victims can be quite serious.

TREATMENT FOR CORAL SNAKE BITES

The venom of the Coral Snake contains a neurotoxin that paralyzes the victim's ability to breathe. Other symptoms include altered mental status, weakness, and partial paralysis. Bite victims often require mechanical or artificial respiration combined with large doses of antivenom. The initial bite is described as painless or very mild, but if left untreated, respiratory failure can occur within a few hours. First aid procedures are similar to the other venomous snakes already discussed. One should keep the victim calm, clean and bandage the bite location, and seek professional medical treatment with a minimum monitoring period of 48 continuous hours. Time is of the essence, so the longer medical treatment is absent, the more likely assisted ventilation will be necessary.

PARTING THOUGHTS ON SNAKES

To summarize, it's clear that venomous snakes should be avoided. However, many snakes, both venomous and not, are killed each year by humans simply because they crossed paths with one another. In many states, it is against the law to kill a non-venomous snake. While we've both come across many snakes during our lives, we've never felt the need to kill one. While we would dispatch a venomous snake if it was in our yard or in close proximity to our family or animals, we've been fortunate in the fact that we've always been able to relocate any non-venomous snakes and simply go around any venomous snakes we've encountered. We've known many people who subscribe to the theory that "the only good snake is a dead snake." (At this point, I (Shawn) fully realize and acknowledge my own hypocrisy, as I will let a snake go, yet kill a spider with a speed and fervor that would make Chuck Norris envious). Unfortunately, this view is detrimental to the surrounding ecosystem, as snakes play a pivotal role in the control of the varmint population. In addition, some snakes such as the non-venomous king snake will actually kill and consume venomous snakes. In the overwhelming majority of encounters, a snake will simply seek to be left alone or will flee the situation altogether. That being said, just because a snake is non-venomous doesn't mean that it does not pose a threat if disturbed or handled. I've caught and handled my share of snakes and fortunately I've only been bitten a handful of times. Even though no venom is involved, the teeth of a non-venomous snake will often puncture the skin and can lead to infection if not cleaned and treated in a timely manner. If you are not well versed in snake identification or you know that you will be in venomous snake habitat, I would strongly advise some sort of protective foot and legwear, such as snake boots and chaps. They will protect your feet, ankles, and legs from a potentially deadly bite. Many loggers and other outdoorsmen incorporate them as part of their daily wear.

Ironically, the last snake I caught was a small ringneck snake that was in my parents' yard. It was only about a foot long and was completely docile as I held it in my hands. I was trying to calm my hysterical mother who automatically assumed it was a rattlesnake, or possibly an anaconda, when I actually said the words "don't worry, these little guys don't bite." Seconds later, he made a liar out of me as he clamped down on a knuckle. While it didn't hurt, I did remove him rather quickly and set him down in the woods behind my parents' house. When I turned and looked at my mother, she was completely pale. Needless to say, she does not share my affinity for reptiles. I've definitely got my work cut out to convince them to simply leave them be, especially when they are non-venomous. In short, if you come across one, just leave it alone. They won't chase you down for the thrill of the hunt, I can assure you (unless it's an ornery Black Racer…but that's another story for another time). As a matter of fact, I walked out one evening a few summers ago to find my cat asleep under my truck with a six-foot long gray rat snake curled up only a couple of feet away from her. My wife asked me if I thought our cat was in danger. I told her that they probably tired each other out comparing stories of catching vermin and that the snake would leave eventually. Sure enough, the next time I checked, the snake had moved on and my cat was fine. Crisis averted.

ALLIGATORS

The final reptile we will cover is the American Alligator. Found in the southeast United States from the coastal Carolinas all the way to Texas, these are the largest reptiles in the United States. Their habitat mainly consists of swampy areas, rivers, streams, lakes, and ponds. In the far south regions of Florida, they are known to cohabitate with the American Crocodile. This is the only place on earth where the two species coexist. Since the American Crocodile is known for its shyness and rarely has interactions with humans, we are not going to feature it as a separate species.

While they definitely look like an oversized lizard, the alligator's closest animal relative is actually a bird. The female American Alligator averages around 8 feet while males come in much longer at around 11 feet on average. Average weight is around 500 pounds, although particularly large male specimens have come in at over 13 feet long and over 1,000 pounds. Their color scheme can be olive, brown,

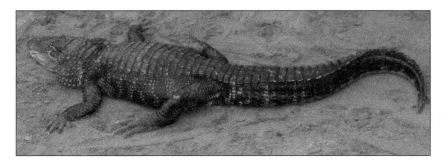

gray, or nearly solid black depending on the type of water they reside in. Their undersides are cream colored and younger alligators have yellowish bands on their tails whereas adults have darker bands on their tails. They are most active around dusk and dawn when they typically feed.

They were once hunted nearly to extinction, yet population numbers have rebounded significantly to the point where there are an estimated 5 million American Alligators alive today, with 1.25 million of those in the state of Florida alone.

ALLIGATOR ATTACK PREVENTION AND TREATMENT

As we have seen with other larger predators, the likelihood of a violent encounter is statistically very rare. However, there still are an average of 10 attacks per year, and there have been around 30 fatalities from 1973-2018. Most of the attacks are when humans have encroached into territory that has been the traditional home of alligators. The reptiles begin to associate humans with food, as pets are often targeted for a quick meal. Couple that with the fact that some people choose to go against nature and feed wild animals, and it's easy to see why there are conflicts between humans and alligators.

When you find yourself in alligator territory, there are several things you can do to minimize your risk. If you are around the banks of a river or pond, keep any animals at least 10 feet away from the water's edge, as alligators are ambush predators and can run as fast as 10 miles an hour for short bursts. Also, avoid swimming in any area that is known to have alligators present, as splashing and loud noises are known to trigger a predatory response. Small children are particularly at risk, as a larger gator can virtually swallow one whole. Many victims have simply disappeared. Avoid walking around coastal areas around dusk and dawn, as these are the alligator's primary feeding hours. If you happen upon baby alligators, immediately leave the area, as the mother is certainly lurking nearby and will act ferociously in defense of her young. If you encounter an alligator trying to cross a street, do not try to assist it. Simply leave it alone and it will go on it's way. Finally, please do not feed them, no matter how small or large they are. What starts out as a novelty can often lead to dangerous consequences, as the animals lose their natural fear of humans. Since alligators can find their way home from up to 100 miles away, relocation is often not an option. As a result, hundreds of alligators are deemed as a "nuisance" every year, with the only available public safety option often resulting in them being killed.

If you do find yourself confronted by an alligator, they will typically growl or huff as a defense mechanism. Slowly walk away from the animal and it will generally leave the area. If you do find yourself being chased by one, run as fast as you can away from it. There has been a long-standing myth that running in a zig-zag pattern will allow you to outpace the alligator. While that may be true, it also highly increases your chances of getting your feet tangled up and taking a fall, which is the last thing you want to do with an angry alligator in pursuit. If you are attacked in the water, go for the animal's eyes and head. Punch, kick, gouge, and hit as fast and furiously as you can. More often than not, the alligator will let go and retreat, but it is by no means a guarantee. Alligators will typically perform a "death roll" with their prey, drowning them and dismembering them to eat later. If you are being attacked by an alligator in the water, you truly are in the fight of your life, so nothing is off limits.

When it comes to treating an alligator attack victim, the first step is to ensure the attack is over and the animal is no longer present. If possible, move the victim to safer ground and perform a visual analysis of wounds. Alligator teeth can puncture and tear, so stopping any arterial bleeding is top priority. Keep the victim as calm as possible and in the event that a limb has been severed, prevent the victim from looking at the wound, as this can trigger panic and lead to even quicker blood loss and shock. Apply a tourniquet if one is present and get the victim to a hospital ASAP. For victims that only have minor cuts or puncture wounds, thoroughly disinfect any open areas, since alligators and the water they reside in are often full of various bacteria that can lead to a serious septic infection if left untreated.

CHAPTER FIVE

WICKED WEATHER

While there seems to be no shortage of animals or insects that pose a threat to those of us who enjoy spending time outdoors, we can't overlook another area of concern: the weather. From bone-chilling cold to intense heat, Mother Nature can certainly throw some curveballs at us. While checking the weather radio before leaving is certainly advised, sometimes the weather can change suddenly, leaving us with little time to react. The purpose of this chapter is to illustrate how to react to these situations.

FROSTBITE

Frostbite is a condition resulting from the freezing of the skin and its underlying tissues. It is most common in the extremities, such as the fingers, toes, nose, ears, cheeks, and chin. Exposed skin is the most vulnerable when out in cold, windy weather. The condition actually takes place in three distinct stages. Frostnip is the most mild condition, with exposure leading to numbness in the skin. Superficial frostbite is the second stage, where the affected skin goes from red to white, with the skin feeling warm. As it progresses, you may feel a burning or stinging sensation coupled with swelling. Fluid-filled blisters may occur in 12-36 hours after rewarming the skin. Deep frostbite is the final and most serious stage. This

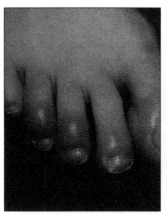
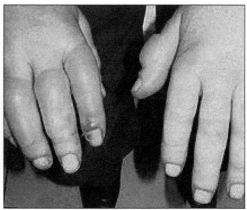

affects both the top and internal layers of skin and tissue, as it turns white or gray. Here, the affected area often goes numb, with joints and muscles refusing to work properly. Large blisters often form within 1-2 days after rewarming. Finally, the affected area turns black and hardens as the top and underlying tissue dies.

The condition takes place in a variety of conditions, such as venturing out into cold weather without proper clothing, remaining in the wind too long (frostbite can occur on exposed in less than 30 minutes), and handling frozen materials or exposed skin coming into contact with cold water. When dressing to go out into an environment that is cold, dress in layers so that you can stay as warm as needed, but can remove layers during periods of exertion such as exercise or strenuous work. Regulating one's temp is critical to avoiding frostbite. Cotton is at the top of the worst choices to wear in this type of environment, as it retains moisture from sweat, snow, etc. Wet clothing clings to the skin and can, in some cases, accelerate the onset of frostbite. Clothing that wicks perspiration away will allow you to stay comfortable and lessen the danger of frostbite. Frostbite is definitely not something to be taken lightly, as it can lead to very serious consequences such as amputation of the affected extremity or infection and gangrene in the affected area.

TREATMENT FOR FROSTBITE

When it comes to first aid procedures, most minor cases can be solved with gradual rewarming and keeping the area clean. For more serious cases, more intensive treatment is required. After rewarming, a doctor may have to loosely wrap the area with sterile dressings, separating fingers and toes as they thaw to protect them. The affected area may be elevated as well to reduce swelling.

Oral medications may be administered for the pain, as well as infection and clot-fighting drugs through an IV to help restore blood flow to the area. In the most severe cases, surgery may be required. This can range from simply removing the dead tissue around the area to full amputation of an extremity or, in worst case scenarios, the entire limb. Thankfully, most occurrences of frostbite are treatable, providing that the victim seek medical care as soon as possible.

HYPOTHERMIA

Simply put, hypothermia is a medical emergency where the body loses heat faster than it can produce it. This leads to the body temperature dropping. It occurs when the body's internal temperature falls below 95 degrees. When this happens, the body begins to shut down, diverting blood flow away from the extremities and towards the internal organs. The heart, nervous system, and other organs cease to function normally. If left untreated, the heart and respiratory system will suffer complete failure, leading to eventual death.

Hypothermia can be caused by a variety of reasons. Exposure to cold weather, over-exertion that leads to heavy sweating and then rapid cooling, and immersion in cold water can lead to hypothermia. There are a variety of symptoms that let you know that your body is in danger. For instance, you may begin shivering, find that you have slurred speech, and slow, shallow breathing. As the condition worsens, you may experience a weakened pulse, lack of coordination, drowsiness, confusion, the stopping of shivering, memory loss, and loss of consciousness. Since the symptoms seem to come on gradually, the victim is often unaware that something is happening until things have progressed to a point of danger. In some instances, the victim's state of confusion may lead them to think that they are actually overheating. Some victims who succumbed to hypothermia have actually been found having shed multiple layers of clothing, only to be overtaken by the elements. It's worth noting that hypothermia is not relegated to just the colder, northern climates. Places like Death Valley and other desert regions cool rapidly after the sun sets, leaving unprepared hikers or outdoors enthusiasts at the mercy of the cold.

Since the effects of hypothermia are gradual and can cause a lot of complications, it is best to prevent them from the offset. When outdoors in cold weather, make sure that your clothing is appropriate for the activity. Wool or modern polypropylene layers are much preferable to cotton. Remember the old adage: cotton kills. If you are going to be exerting a lot of energy, such as hiking or jogging, ensure that you are wearing layers that wick away moisture from the inside out. This will help regulate your temperature and ensure that you don't become wet on your base layers and then begin to lose body heat as you cool off. Avoid exposure to water, as it can rapidly cause heat loss from any exposed skin. It's also advisable to keep a toque or hat on, as the majority of heat is lost through the head. Wind can also be a danger, as it can blow away the thin layer of heat on our skin, causing the body to drop in temperature. With the proper clothing and precautions, enjoying the outdoors in the colder months can be as enjoyable as the warmer months. Just ensure that you are adequately prepared, and consider adding an emergency blanket (sometimes referred to as a space blanket) to your kit, as you can wrap up a hypothermia victim in it to prevent further heat loss.

TREATMENT FOR HYPOTHERMIA

If you encounter someone with hypothermia or find yourself starting to exhibit the symptoms, there are steps you can take to treat the condition. First of all, get the victim indoors and remove any wet clothing and dry the person off. Gradually begin to warm the victim, starting with the person's core (if outdoors, the best course of action may be skin-to-skin contact). Take care that you don't immerse the victim in warm water or start warming extremities first. This can lead to shock and possible heart conditions as the body reacts to the sudden warming. If the pulse slows or the person ceases to breathe, initiate CPR and contact emergency medical services. If the person begins to come around, you can give warm drinks such as tea, making sure to avoid caffeine and alcohol-based drinks.

HEAT CRAMPS

Heat cramps are painful muscle cramps that occur during activity in a hot environment. They normally involve muscles spasming or jerking involuntarily. A lack of electrolytes may be a contributor to the condition as well as they are lost through the process of sweating. Heat cramps are typically short in duration, but may be the first sign of a more serious condition called heat exhaustion. First aid for heat cramps involves resting in a cool place and replacing lost fluids through drinking water or sports drinks such as Gatorade, which replace lost electrolytes.

Gentle stretching exercises can also provide relief. Heat cramps are common in sports such as football where practices and games take place in very hot, humid conditions. The condition can take place when performing work in hot environments or strenuous activities such as hiking, biking, running, etc.

HEAT EXHAUSTION

The next step of heat illness is heat exhaustion. This is a condition characterized by heavy sweating and an elevated pulse. It most often takes place after exposure to high temperatures and humid conditions. Working environments that are hot and humid and prolonged exercise sessions are the most common triggers for heat exhaustion. In northwest Georgia, we have heat and high humidity for the majority of the year. Every summer, there are multiple cases of heat exhaustion among school athletes and factory workers. I've spent nearly 15 years working in and around carpet mills, and the conditions inside during the summer can be stifling, to put it mildly. Our employees are encouraged to dress appropriately and stay hydrated. Large industrial fans are placed in many areas in order to keep the air flowing, but it's still beyond miserable at times.

Along with excessive sweating, the victim may experience cool and moist skin, faintness, goosebumps, dizziness, fatigue, muscle cramps, nausea, and a headache. First aid for this condition begins with stopping the activity and allowing the victim to rest in a cooler place. Loosen any restrictive clothing and help the victim to drink cool water or sports drinks to replace lost electrolytes.

HEAT STROKE

The most severe of the heat illnesses is heat stroke. This is a condition where the body overheats, with internal temperatures rising to 104 degrees. It is brought on by prolonged exposure to high temperatures or extreme physical exertion. This condition can be life threatening and often requires emergency treatment. Left unchecked, it can lead to brain, heart, kidney, and muscle damage. The condition only worsens the longer treatment is delayed. Symptoms to look for are core body temps of 104 degrees or higher, altered mental state, confusion, agitation, slurred speech, irritability, and seizures. In addition, the victim often stops sweating, with the skin being hot and dry to the touch. Nausea and vomiting are common, as is rapid breathing, elevated heart rate, and a severe headache.

TREATMENT FOR HEAT STROKE

First aid for heat stroke involves getting the victim to professional medical care as soon as possible. If that is not an option, move the person to a shaded area and remove excess clothing. Then, put the victim in cool water and/or spray the victim with water to begin the cooling process. Putting ice packs or cold towels on the head, neck, groin, and armpits can also aid in bringing down the victim's internal temperature. If the person is conscious, administer fluids to help bring down internal temps. Be sure to monitor the victim while they are drinking, because if they were to slip unconscious, the victim could choke on the liquids. Heat stroke is a serious condition, but thankfully can be avoided by a little preparation. Try to avoid strenuous activity during the hottest part of the day. Stay hydrated and wear loose-fitting clothing and be aware of the onset of symptoms in yourself or others. The faster a heat-related illness is addressed, the quicker and simpler the recovery.

SUNBURN

There's probably very few people who haven't experienced a sunburn at some point in their life. Simply put, a sunburn is the condition that you experience when your skin has been exposed to the sun's rays unprotected for a prolonged period of time.

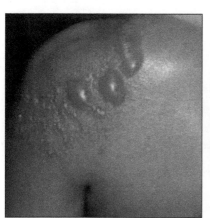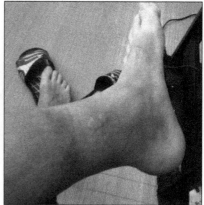

Examples range from too much time at the beach without proper sunscreen to suffering the effects of snow reflection, where the sun's rays reflect off the snow. The typical symptoms are redness of the skin along with pain and sometimes swelling. If the burn is severe enough, the skin may begin to blister and in the most severe cases, the victim may experience nausea, headache, weakness, and a feverish feeling complete with chills. Within a few days of overexposure, the skin will begin to itch and peel as the body begins to rid itself of the skin cells damaged by the sun.

TREATMENT FOR SUNBURN

Treating sunburn is fairly simple. Cold compresses or a cool oatmeal bath can help soothe the burning sensation, as well as various topical ointments. The most effective are those containing menthol, aloe, calendula or camphor. Apple cider vinegar in a bath is very effective, as is lavender and/or peppermint oil. In addition, ibuprofen and naproxen can often relieve swelling and pain associated with sunburn. Try to avoid scratching the skin as the peeling begins. Excessive scratching can break the surface of the skin near the burn and sometimes results in an infection.

Prevention is key when it comes to avoiding sunburn. If you know that you will be active when the sun is out, ensure that you are wearing an adequate sunscreen and definitely re-apply as needed. Activities that result in a lot of sweating may need to see periodic re-application. Consider the fact that even on partly cloudy days, the sun's rays shine through, so take proper precautions then as well. Also, consider wearing a hat or other head-covering and light-colored, loose-fitting, long sleeve shirts and pants. The more you cover, the less skin is exposed to the sun's damaging rays.

DEHYDRATION

As its name implies, dehydration is a condition where the body is using or losing more fluid than it is taking in. This condition can occur during times of extreme exertion where fluid is lost through sweating, especially in hot and humid environments where sweat does not evaporate quickly. Symptoms of dehydration include extreme thirst, less frequent urination, dark-colored urine, overall fatigue, dizziness, and confusion.

TREATMENT FOR DEHYDRATION

First aid for minor cases of dehydration include taking a break and drinking water or sports drinks to replace lost electrolytes. Most cases of dehydration are minor and resolve themselves through fluid replenishment. However, in more serious cases, hospitalization may be required and intravenous fluids introduced. To prevent the onset of dehydration, ensure you are drinking enough water during times of exertion and high humidity. Don't wait until you start to feel thirsty, either, as dehydration can already be setting in by the time you do.

WATER HAZARDS

Sometimes the best way to cool off on a summer hike and relax is to take a stroll through a cool, gentle creek or take a dip in the lake or the ocean. However, bodies of water, regardless of their size, can all have inherent risks associated with them. In the United States alone, there are over 3,500 non-boating related drownings each year. Many of these are the result of people not knowing how to swim properly and panicking. In addition, there are people who are in top shape and great swimmers that sometimes fall victim to drowning. One example that hits close to home is that of a classmate of my son. At the time, he was 13 and hiking in Colorado with his grandmother over spring break. Both were in peak physical condition and were familiar with the terrain, as they had been hiking the trails in the area for many years. They were attempting to cross a small river that was swollen due to recent heavy rains. At some point, one of them slipped and fell into the fast-moving water and knocked the other one over. Rescue crews searched the area for nearly a month before finding their bodies. It was a devastating shock to the whole school and community, and a dark reminder that water has a power of its own and is to be respected.

In addition to inland threats, the ocean provides a series of dangers as well. Rip tides and strong currents can drag a person out to sea within minutes and are very difficult to overcome. Even the strongest swimmer will tire eventually and can succumb to the sea. Bodies of water should be enjoyed, but done so safely. Always ensure that if you are crossing a body of water, you have a proper foothold and know if there are any sudden depth changes. One slip on a wet rock can send a person tumbling, possibly incurring a broken bone or head injury. If hiking alone, this could prove fatal in some cases. When your outdoor adventures take you near water, always make sure that those in your party can swim and that no one wanders off alone. If going to the beach, take the time to read the warning signs about rip tides and currents, and how to escape them should you find yourself caught up in one. Reading and understanding how nature works could literally save your life.

WILDFIRES

Every year, hundreds of thousands of acres of forest and open land are consumed by wildfires. Entire communities and small towns have been destroyed by these fires. Sometimes they are caused by a lightning strike and other times they are caused due to human factors such as a camp fire not being fully extinguished or arson. Regardless of the cause, they can get out of control in a hurry, threatening both human and animal habitats. If you find yourself outdoors in the proximity of one of these fires, ensure that it is not an immediate threat to the area you are in.

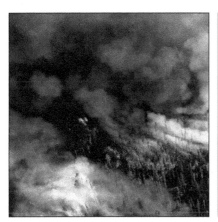 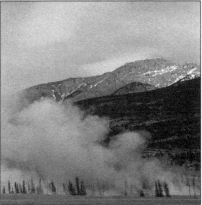

Wildfires can spread rapidly and jump small bodies of water, so just because there is a creek or river nearby doesn't mean you are guaranteed safety. Also consider the harmful smoke in the air. People with breathing issues are at high risk from the smoke and its contents, as it can blow several miles from the actual fire. In addition, when fires overcome roadways, traffic can become a nightmare, as people try to turn around and flee the area while first responders and fire crews attempt to get in so they can fight it. As with other types of weather hazards, checking the conditions of the area you will be travelling to beforehand can save you and your family or friends a lot of grief over finding yourself at the mercy of mother nature.

LIGHTNING

Most all of us have been taught to seek shelter when a thunderstorm blows up in the sky. However, sometimes lightning can seem to come out of nowhere, posing a definite threat to someone who is exposed outdoors. Thousands of people are struck by lightning annually. Thankfully, only a fraction of the strikes result in a fatality. However, the survivors of lightning attacks often have lingering effects from the experience.

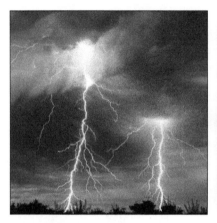 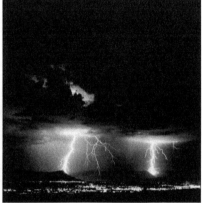

When lightning strikes a person, it rarely travels through the body. Instead, it travels over the body in what is referred to as a "flashover." Fatalities from lightning strikes most often are a result of cardiac arrest that is brought on due to the massive electrical discharge. As the electricity travels over the body, it turns sweat and rainwater into a scalding steam. It also can transfer objects such as jewelry and car keys into red hot items that can leave serious burns. In addition, clothing can be shredded or even lit on fire by the massive heat from the lightning bolt. Often times, the victim's footwear and socks are blown off as the lightning passes over.

Oddly enough, many lightning strike survivors don't have any memory of being struck. Physical or neurological evidence can be plentiful, though. Some victims will exhibit both an entry and exit wound where the electric current entered and left them. The result can be scarring in the form of the outlines of ruptured blood vessels under the skin in spider web-like patterns. Neurological effects can be even more serious. A lightning strike may allow electrical current to directly enter the brain, essentially cooking brain cells. This can result in memory loss, trouble concentrating, blown-out eardrums, and severe headaches. These effects can be residual, lasting decades after the strike took place.

TREATMENT FOR A LIGHTNING STRIKE

First aid for lightning strikes should always start with calling 911. A common reaction to a lightning strike is cardiac arrest. If the victim is not breathing, CPR should be administered immediately after the victim is moved to a safe location. There is no risk of electrocution, as the charge has already left the body. If there are burns present, do not try to remove burned clothing, as it may lead to skin loss. If the victim begins to show signs of shock, lay them down, with their head slightly lower than the torso and legs. Once at a hospital, medical personnel can examine the victim and determine the severity of both physical and neurological trauma.

Reducing the likelihood of being struck by lightning is fairly simple. Checking the weather conditions before embarking on an outdoor adventure can alert you to any possibility of a thunderstorm occurring in the area. However, as many of us have experienced during the spring and summer, pop-up thunderstorms can appear with little to no warning. The CDC recommends the 30-30 rule. This rule advises to start counting to 30 when you see lightning flash. If you hear thunder before you reach 30, it's advisable to go indoors. Delay any activities for at least 30 minutes after the last clap of thunder. If shelter is not available, crouch low, with as little of your body as possible touching the ground. Definitely do not seek shelter under a large tree, as lightning is often attracted to the tallest object in an area. Statistically, you only have a 1 in 500,000 chance of being struck by lighting. While those odds are definitely in your favor, it is still very advisable to minimize those chances as much as possible.

CHAPTER SIX

WILDERNESS FIRST AID BASICS

When enjoying the great outdoors, it is essential to have the right gear on hand. Included in the term "gear" should be the knowledge and applicable skill sets of basic wilderness first aid. For the purposes of this book, we will discuss the absolute basic minimum. If you will be spending a lot of time in the outdoors or will be responsible for the safety and well being of others, it would be very advisable to get your certification in wilderness first aid from an organization such as the Red Cross. Their courses are taught nationwide and you will likely be able to find one available near you.

The first skill that you should be proficient in would be the cleaning and bandaging of minor cuts and scrapes. Your first aid kit should have the adequate alcohol wipes and bandaids to clean a cut or puncture wound and bandage it to keep infection from setting in. Steri-strips for a more serious laceration are part of any good first aid kit. A basic first aid salve (see the appendix for a recipe) is always a part of our kits to keep infection at bay and help with pain and inflammation. Next, you should be proficient in treating minor sprains, such as an ankle or wrist sprain from a fall. Your kit should contain athletic gauze to wrap and stabilize a sprain injury and perhaps an ice pack to help minimize swelling.

Another valuable skill is being able to deal with a bite or sting from an insect or animal. If the victim is allergic, knowing how to administer an Epipen injection and an antihistamine is crucial. For people not allergic, knowing how to clean and remove a stinger is necessary. A topical cream or ointment can help to minimize the discomfort. For something as serious as a venomous snake bite, keeping a victim calm and collected and calling for help is critical.

For other serious injuries, such as broken bones, stabilizing the victim will be paramount until it's determined whether or not they can be safely moved. Covering and cleaning the wound should be done if possible until professional help arrives. Keeping the victim calm and not allowing them to go into shock or suffer extreme blood loss is important. Should medical help be unreachable or cannot get to your location quickly enough, determine whether or not the victim can be safely moved via an improvised stretcher. If that is not an option, a splint carried in your first aid kit can help stabilize the break enough to get the victim to a location where medical professionals can meet you.

In the event that an injury leads to excessive blood loss, having a suitable tourniquet in your kit can be life saving. Proper application of a tourniquet can buy the victim time to be transported to professional medical help. No wilderness kit should be without a tourniquet. It is one of the most essential pieces of gear to carry. Blood loss can quickly turn a minor injury into a serious one in very short order. Having a blood clotting agent in the form of a trauma clotting sponge is essential for controlling bleeding. Applying the sponge and securing it can prevent further blood loss and minimize the chance of infection settling into an open wound.

Finally, knowing the basics of CPR and rescue breathing can be instrumental in saving the life of a person suffering from cardiac arrest. Since most of us won't have an AED (Automated External Defibrillator) handy, knowing the proper hand placement and chest compression counts can help keep a victim alive until help arrives. We advise having a CPR mask as part of your wilderness first aid kit, as it allows the caregiver to avoid direct contact with the victim's mouth. Since cardiac arrest victims sometimes vomit as CPR is applied, the mouth shield can keep any bodily fluids from coming into contact with the caregiver's mouth. Be aware that administering CPR will often result in accidentally broken ribs, as the chest compressions are so close to the rib cage. This is a small price to be paid for saving a life. If this does happen, there are laws that protect the caregiver. Often referred to as Good Samaritan laws, they protect and encourage qualified individuals to administer this lifesaving course of action without fear of legal recourse should a rib be broken during the process.

A quality wilderness first aid kit should also contain a variety of medicines to deal with other issues that may arise during time spent outdoors. At a minimum, a kit should contain pain relievers such as ibuprofen and acetaminophen for headaches and muscle pain. Stomach and diarrhea relief medications should also be included, because left unchecked, these conditions can often lead to dehydration. Antihistamines in the form of pills and creams are useful to counteract allergic reactions to plant or animal encounters.

Burn gel is also a great addition to your kit. I've witnessed firsthand the damage that can be done by reaching into a campfire after accidentally dropping a mess kit into it while heating up an evening meal. It happened to a good friend of mine and his pointer and middle finger were nearly fused together as a result of mindlessly reaching into the campfire as his mess kit fell off a log while heating up some stew. I had to apply burn cream to his fingers and wrapped them together with non-stick gauze for the duration of the trip. The first aid performed kept him from any further damage, and regular doses of ibuprofen kept pain down to a minimum level considering the extent of his injury. We wound up getting through the rest of the trip with no further incidents and the wound area was cleaned and treated by his doctor the day after we returned home. He took a while to heal, as the burn affected multiple skin layers, but could have been much worse had treatment not been administered at the time of the injury. Burn gel comes in small packets, so there's no reason not to have several in your first aid kit.

Next, a pair of tweezers, a fresnel lens (for magnification), and a small flashlight should be included in your first aid kit. This will aid in the removal of ticks and splinters and allow you or a friend to illuminate the area. A good antibiotic cream such as Neosporin or a First Aid Salve can be invaluable to ensure that a wound stays infection free, as well as alcohol pads to clean the area before treatment is applied. Finally, some moleskin should be included to help with any areas that become blistered as a result of friction, most often on the feet.

It's obvious that you cannot plan for every injury or contingency that may occur during an outdoor trip. However, proper planning along with an adequately-stocked first aid kit can ensure that any problems that arise can be dealt with in a manner that protects the victim and minimizes any long term effects of an injury. As stated earlier, avoid the temptation to simply buy one of the small, travel-sized kits you find in the pharmacy section. Use discretion, and plan for the encounters that you deem most likely and plan accordingly. A well thought out first aid kit can be worth its weight in gold should it be needed in the event of an injury.

Finally, if you are not certain about how to handle anything beyond a minor cut or sprain, take a certification course. The Red Cross has classes in most major cities for the basics of first aid and how to perform CPR. These classes typically last a few hours and include both written testing and simulations using CPR mannequins. They are very thorough and well worth the time and money spent. Often times, your workplace may offer these classes, so check with your Human Resources or EHS department and find out what may be available. Another good source of training would be your city or county C.E.R.T. (community emergency response team). I personally am a member of the Walker County, Georgia C.E.R.T. and joined largely because of the various training classes that are available. Nicole is a member of the Pacific County, Washington C.E.R.T. and assists with training there. Also consider that these skills are somewhat perishable, so be sure to get recertified periodically. It's some of the best knowledge that a person can have, and it may just save a life.

CHAPTER SEVEN

PLANNING YOUR NEXT ADVENTURE

As was mentioned in the beginning of the book, most problems that arise during a trip into the outdoors can be minimized or eliminated altogether by prior planning. Just like you wouldn't jet off to Disney World without researching ticket prices and hotel room rates, you shouldn't embark on a trip into the outdoors without at least some amount of planning. While this doesn't mean that you need to sit down and map every step you take while on your excursion, you should be somewhat prepared for any issues that pop up while you are out.

For instance, if you are planning anything from a quick daytime hike to a multi-day camping trip, let at least one person know when you are leaving, where you are going, and approximately when you should return. This will allow someone to know when it's time to get concerned and check on your well-being. If you are in a somewhat of a remote location, it will also allow search teams to have a general idea of where to start searching. If you've become injured, this could literally be the difference between life and death. Also, if you will be going on your adventure solo, you should consider a GPS device that allows you to send out a distress signal should you become lost or incapacitated. Cell phones are great to have, but often times in the outdoors reception can be unreliable or the battery may run out at the worst possible time. It's a good idea to have a backup means of contacting help. Prices have fallen in the last few years, and the technology has advanced to where these devices can fit easily into your pack or pocket and be deployed by the simple press of a button, sending location and other relevant data to search and rescue teams.

If you are going to be out with a group, note in advance any pre-existing health issues or bodily limitations that may complicate the activity. Plan in advance the route you are to take, and ensure that the terrain is conducive to everyone in your party. When it comes to medical issues, simply knowing if someone is prone to seizures, allergic to insect venom, or has a heart condition can allow you to temper expectations and ensure that person does not overexert themselves. It also allows you a heads-up should an emergency arise. By now, you should definitely see the importance of carrying an adequate first aid kit that is tailored to the situation, such as the addition of an Epipen for someone allergic to bee stings.

Ensure beforehand that you have enough food and water for the duration of your trip. Food should always be in a container that is not easily opened and that can be kept out of the reach of curious forest critters. When it comes to water, I've learned firsthand that the water sources marked on a map are not always guaranteed, and I've had times that I've basically been purifying a mud puddle just to have potable water. Always ensure that you have a way to purify water because no matter how clear it looks, it always has the potential to make you sick. I also like to carry a collapsible five gallon container that I fill up with purified water to use as camp water. That allows me to keep my drinking containers full, as well as being able to cook and wash my gear later on. Before leaving the next morning, I make sure to top off all my drinking containers and use any leftover water to ensure that any fires from the previous night are completely extinguished.

If a multi-day trip is indeed taking place, ensure that hygiene does not become an issue. While there are restroom and shower facilities at some campsites, more often than not, you are on your own when in the backcountry. I carry lightweight, fast drying wash towels and biodegradable soap in my gear and have taken many a shower or bath in fast moving creeks, but more often than not, I use unscented baby wipes or something similar to clean myself. A pack of these for each member of your party can keep people from the "nasty and gross" feelings that comes from a day or two without a shower. They are lightweight and come in styles that are biodegradable.

A check of the weather for the upcoming day or days to come is also a prudent move. While the weather can often change without warning, having a general idea about upcoming conditions can assist you with making sure you and your party are equipped properly in regards to clothing and gear. Every year, hikers are rescued after spending an unexpected night off the trail due to getting lost or running out of daylight. Having the proper clothing and gear can keep an inconvenience from turning into a life-threatening situation. It should go without saying that regardless if you are on a day hike or a week-long expedition, you should have the proper emergency gear on hand. We covered this in chapter one, and a checklist can be found in the appendix section in the back of the book.

If you are planning an overnight or multi-night stay, ensure that your shelter is adequate. If tent camping, ensure that your tent is large enough for the occupant (s) and gear and that it is rated for that season. Lots of people have spent a miserable night in a bargain-basement, warm-weather only tent when they should have brought along a more appropriate model. Shelter is not an area to skimp on. Cheap tents tend to tear and leak, which can turn a pleasant trip into a nightmare quickly. As with all of your gear, ensure that your shelter is up to the task. The days of big, bulky tents is a thing of the past. Modern backpacking tents can weigh next to nothing and can provide a safe haven from the cold and rain outside. The same logic applies to sleeping bags. Make sure that what you have is rated for where you are and what time of the year it is.

Knowledge of the area you will be in is crucial as well. What type of terrain will you be working with? What type of plant life and wildlife are you likely to encounter? Are there multiple ways to and from your destination should the main trail be blocked or closed? Are there landmarks that you can orient your direction by? Asking simple questions like these will allow you to be better mentally prepared for the unknown. Know what level of gear each member in your party is able to comfortably carry. A great way to ruin an outdoor experience for kids (and some adults) is to overload a backpack that has to be carried along a 3 mile trail to the campsite.

The less you leave to chance, the better off you will be. The old adage of "proper preparation prevents poor performance" is quite true. A little more time spent planning on the front end will allow you to enjoy your outdoor experience more and be able to react to any changes with a better level of preparedness.

CHAPTER EIGHT

IN CLOSING

I hope that you, the reader, have found this book to be informative and beneficial, and hopefully a little entertaining as well. I had a wonderful time researching and writing it along with Nicole. She is a wealth of knowledge and a great friend to boot! Enjoying the outdoors is something we should all do from time to time. Nature itself can be not only refreshing to the soul, but good for us physically as well. For instance, I would much rather hike a few miles in the woods than to run a few boring miles on the treadmill. There's something about being in the outdoors that just feels right. If you follow Nicole on Facebook or Twitter, you've likely seen some of the articles she has posted on the link between spending more time outdoors and better mental health in both children and adults. It's no surprise that many people find spending time in nature to be somewhat of a "reset button" for their stressful lives.

I hope that you have seen that, while there are certain threats that are inherent with being out in nature, a little bit of pre-planning can reduce the anxiety and severity of them. The purpose of this book is not to focus on the things that may affect us negatively while outdoors. Rather, the intent is to show how to identify, treat, and move on from the problems we might encounter with as little disruption as possible, and should a life-threatening event occur, to deal with it as calmly and rationally as possible. Statistically, an event such as an animal bite or lightning strike is very low, but if you happen to find yourself being that 1 out of 10,000 who is the victim, having the knowledge to identify and begin self-treatment can be lifesaving.

Finally, if you enjoy the great outdoors, I encourage you to find someone who doesn't get out much and introduce them to what they are missing. They may find that a whole new world is at their fingertips. We are truly blessed in this country to have access to so many wonderful areas, both public and private. There are federal and state parks, along with many privately-funded preserves. I'm fortunate that in my area, I have two wonderful privately-funded areas to enjoy, the Reflection Riding Arboretum and Nature Center and Audubon Acres, are within 30 minutes of my house and offer acres of pristine wilderness and walking trails. More details are in the appendix if you are in this area and want to learn more. My hope is that you and your family and friends take advantage of what is offered. Go for a hike. Take a swim. Take your kids on a camping trip. Find that hidden trout stream and test your fly fishing skills. Venture out on a cold fall morning and try your hand at putting some venison in the freezer. The outdoors is beckoning.......go answer that call!

APPENDIX &
RESOURCE GUIDE

This section of the book is designed to provide you with information regarding where to find the different gear and resources to make your time in the outdoors more enjoyable and you more prepared for any uncertainties that may arise. At the end of this section, you will find several blank, lined pages that are provided for you to make your own notes and checklists.

KNIVES / MULTITOOLS

Knives have been an essential tool for humans from the earliest recorded history. I personally never leave home without at least one knife on me. Here are several modern companies that make knives and multitools. There is something for every budget listed below:

MORA KNIVES
https://www.industrialrev.com/morakniv

LT WRIGHT KNIVES
https://ltwrightknives.com/

BARK RIVER KNIVES
https://www.barkriverknives.com/index/

SPYDERCO KNIVES
https://www.spyderco.com/

BENCHMADE KNIVES
https://www.benchmade.com/

LEATHERMAN MULTITOOLS
https://www.leatherman.com/

GERBER KNIVES AND MULTITOOLS
https://www.gerbergear.com/

GEP III HANDMADE KNIVES
https://www.facebook.com/gep3handmadeknives/

BUCK KNIVES
https://www.buckknives.com/

VICTORINOX SWISS ARMY KNIVES
https://www.swissarmy.com/us/en/Products/Swiss-Army-Knives/c/SAK

ESEE KNIVES
https://www.eseeknives.com/

ZT KNIVES
https://zt.kaiusaltd.com/

KERSHAW KNIVES
https://kershaw.kaiusaltd.com/

CASE CUTLERY
https://caseknives.com/

COLD STEEL KNIVES
https://www.coldsteel.com/

SOG KNIVES
https://www.sogknives.com/

SMOKY MOUNTAIN KNIFE WORKS
https://www.smkw.com/

BASIC EMERGENCY FIELD KIT
AS RECOMMENDED BY NICOLE APELIAN

The following items make up a checklist for a basic emergency field kit that should be on your person at all times when outdoors, and should all fit in one small bag you carry with you. You can add or substitute additional items to customize it to your specific needs. The items can be found at the retailers listed in the sections below, such as Wazoo Survival Gear and Five Star Gear.

Check off items as you obtain them. This article by Nicole has links to where you can get these items inexpensively: https://www.nicoleapelian.com/blog/basic-emergency-field-kit/

FIRE
- [ ] Ferro rod
- [ ] Lighter
- [ ] Fire starting tinder
- [ ] Fresnel lens

SIGNALING
- [ ] Map compass
- [ ] Emergency whistle
- [ ] Signal mirror
- [ ] Bright neon flag / clothing
- [ ] Small flashlight with extra batteries

WATER
- [ ] Steel water bottle kit with nesting cup for cooking
- [ ] Water bags
- [ ] Water purification tablets
- [ ] Sawyer Mini water filter

SHELTER
- [ ] Paracord - at least 20'
- [ ] Wire saw
- [ ] Emergency rain poncho
- [ ] Emergency tarp / shelter sheet
- [ ] Mylar blanket

FOOD PROCUREMENT

- [ ] 28 gauge brass snare wire
- [ ] Fishing line and hooks

OTHER

- [ ] Mora Knife (or other type)
- [ ] Extra small knife / saw combo
- [ ] Small sewing kit
- [ ] Local area map

FIRST AID / MEDICAL

- [ ] Emergency medication (anti-diarrheal, aspirin, Ibuprofen, Benadryl, prescription medication)
- [ ] 3 Bandaids (minimum)
- [ ] 2 Butterfly closures (minimum)
- [ ] First aid salve
- [ ] RevMedX and/or SWAT-T tourniquet
- [ ] Chito-Sam and/or Israeli Bandage

SIGNALING

If you are going to be in the outdoors, alone or in a group, it's always good to have some sort of signaling or communication device besides your cell phone. Below are a few suggestions that go beyond the minimum field kit checklist above. If you are going to be in a very remote area, I would advise having multiple options to signal for help.

FLARES

Lightweight and easy to use, flares are a very effective way to broadcast your location to rescue teams, especially at night. Keeping road flares in your vehicle can help avoid accidents should your vehicle become disabled. Orion is one of the most trusted names in safety and signaling methods. **http://www.orionsignals.com**

SMOKE GRENADES

While it may seem a little dramatic and over the top, smoke grenades can actually be very helpful when signaling for help in the daytime. In some mountainous regions, fog and low cloud cover can allow the smoke from a signal fire to go unnoticed. Dense cover can also hinder the use of flares. However, colored smoke is easily visible from the air and can help guide in rescue teams. I would caution to stay away from the firework variety, as they can fail and may not have the range necessary to be seen. **https://ustacticalsupply.com/smokegrenades.aspx**

EMERGENCY LOCATOR BEACONS

Beacons can be as simple as location markers or advanced enough to allow the user to send status updates to loved ones. Since there are so many versions available, here is a website that breaks down the various models by strengths and weaknesses. **https://www.outdoorgearlab.com/topics/camping-and-hiking/best-personal-locator-beacon**

FLASHLIGHTS

A quality, high lumen flashlight can be visible for long distances, especially at night. Here are some links to some recommended brands of flashlights. Be sure to have at least one set of extra batteries before embarking on your excursion.

SUREFIRE

https://www.surefire.com/

STREAMLIGHT

https://www.streamlight.com/

TRU SPEC

https://www.truspec.com/accessories/misc-equipment/ts-hp-80-led-flashlight

OLIGHT

https://olightworld.com/

MAGLITE

https://maglite.com/

SIX COMMON MEDICINAL PLANTS AND LICHENS FOR USE IN THE FIELD

Many more plants, lichens, fungi and their uses can be found at:
www.nicoleapelian.com/blog/about-herbal-tinctures-and-healing-salves/

The following are easy to find plants that are considered good for field use. A plant identification guide is recommended.

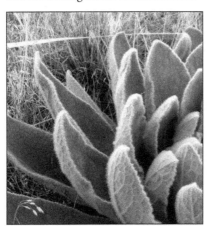 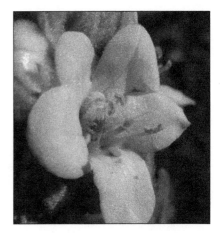

MULLEIN
With leaves that work well as toilet paper, mullein *(Verbascum Thapsus)* tea is also known to treat respiratory conditions such as asthma, bronchitis, allergies, sore throats and coughs. A poultice (a paste you can make with herbs mixed with water) can be put on rashes, bruises, arthritis, cold sores, and hemorrhoids.

PLANTAIN
My kids and I always pick plantain *(Plantago Sp.)* if we get a bite or sting from an insect and then put the chewed leaf on our sting. It works very well for us! We use it externally for swollen joints, sore muscles, sprains, insect bites

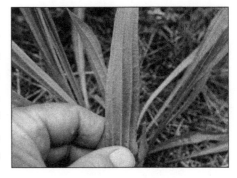

and stings (removes itch and pain), and snakebites. The tannins in it help stop bleeding. We drink the tea for diarrhea and intestinal worms. *Plantago major & Plantago lanceolata*

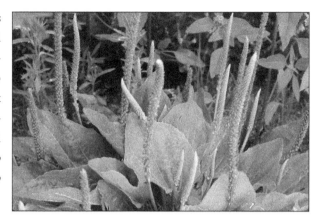

STINGING NETTLE

Stinging Nettle *(Urtica dioica)* delicious plant to eat when cooked it is known for allergy relief, as an anti-inflammatory, and to help with bladder infections, joint pain, eczema and arthritis.

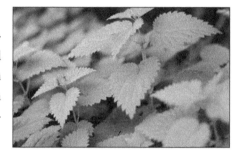

OLD MAN'S BEARD LICHEN

Old Man's Beard *(Usnea Spp.)* lichen, which can be identified by its rubber-band like inner strand, is known as an excellent antifungal, antibacterial and antiviral. It is said to work on staph infections, athlete's foot, strep throat, respiratory tract infections, skin infections, UTIs and more. I have put it directly on wounds in the field and used a strong tea brew of this and yarrow to stop infection in wounds.

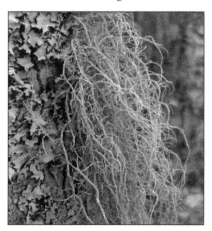

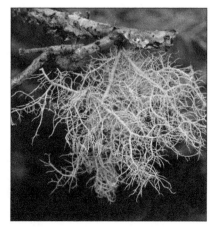

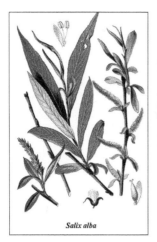

Salix alba

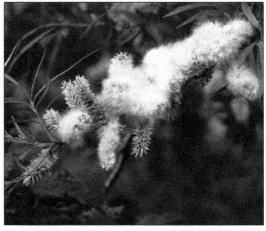

WILLOW

Willow bark *(Salix spp.)* contains salicin, which is nature's aspirin. Do not give this to people who are bleeding heavily as it is an anticoagulant. It is good for pain and as an anti-inflammatory. It can also bring down fever. I chew on the end of a small branch when in need of aspirin in the field. You can also make a tea from the inner bark.

YARROW

Yarrow *(Achillea millefolium)* is known as a great antibacterial and I use it for wounds. It is also a coagulant so it helps stop bleeding when put on a wound (use the leaves and/or flowers). It is also known for helping ear infections, relieving fevers, shortening the duration of cold and flu, helping improve relaxation during illness, and relieving cramps associated with hormones or illness. Applied topically, it is said to help with skin itching, rash, infection or other issues.

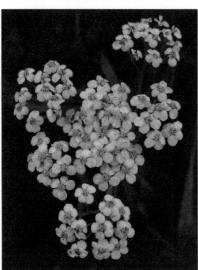

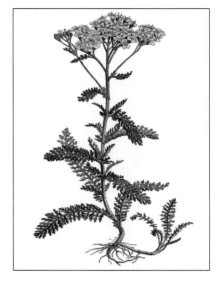

DR. NICOLE'S NATURAL RECIPES FOR PAIN RELIEF

Nicole's Bite/Rash/Sting Salve: Plantain (Plantago sp.), Calendula, Lavender Essential Oil, Tea Tree Essential Oil and Vitamin E in Organic Olive Oil and Beeswax.

First Aid Salve: Yarrow, Arnica, Calendula, Plantain, Cottonwood Buds, Vitamin E, and Lavender Essential Oil in Organic Olive Oil and Beeswax.

Nicole's salves are available on her website (www.nicoleapelian.com). If you would like to make a salve at home, here are her directions:

1. Infuse dry herbs into organic olive oil for 6-8 weeks in a glass jar. I fill the jar ½ full of dried herbs and then fill with oil almost to the top and cover. Mark the date and type of herbal oil using a label. If you remember it's good to shake it every once in a while.

2. Once the medicine has infused into the oil (about 2 months time), strain with cheesecloth and discard the plant material.

3. Measure your various infused medicinal oils and put into a double boiler on low heat. Add beeswax in a 1:4 ratio (1 part beeswax to 4 parts oil). So for 16 oz of herbal oil, add 4 oz of beeswax.

4. Stir until the beeswax is melted, then add ¼ tsp Vitamin E per 16 oz of oil and 20 drops of each essential oil.

5. Pour into your tins or jars and allow time to harden. Label.

NATURAL BUG AND TICK REPELLENT SPRAY

Use witch hazel in a glass spray bottle as your base and add the following essential oils (you need not add them all but this is a list of ones you can add and mix together). I use 60 drops total of the oils I want for 8 oz of spray. Apply every 2 hours.

Essential Oils that work to repel insects:
• Lemongrass
• Lemon Eucalyptus
• Lavender
• Rosemary
• Thyme
• Tea Tree
• Geranium
• Citronella
• Peppermint
• Basil
• Vetiver
• Oregano

You can find a good selection of essential oils at your local Whole Foods store. (https://www.wholefoodsmarket.com/)

HERE IS A LINK TO NICOLE'S SALVES AND TINCTURES:

https://www.nicoleapelian.com/blog/about-herbal-tinctures-and-healing-salves/

GEAR SELECTION

The following retailers will help you put together all the gear you need for your next outdoor adventure.

FIVE STAR GEAR
https://www.5ivestargear.com/

CABELA'S
https://www.cabelas.com/

BASS PRO SHOPS
https://www.basspro.com/

GANDER OUTDOORS (FORMERLY GANDER MOUNTAIN)
https://www.ganderoutdoors.com/

ACADEMY SPORTS
https://www.academy.com/

SPORTSMAN'S GUIDE
https://www.sportsmansguide.com/

SPORTSMAN'S WAREHOUSE
https://www.sportsmanswarehouse.com/

CAROLINA READINESS:
https://carolinareadiness.com/

TENNESSEE READINESS
https://www.tennesseereadiness.com/

P5 PREPAREDNES:
https://www.p5preparedness.com/

WAZOO SURVIVAL GEAR
https://www.wazoosurvivalgear.com/

EMERGENCY ESSENTIAL:
https://www.beprepared.com/

SURVIVAL DISPATCH
http://www.survivaldispatch.com/

TRUSPEC
https://www.truspec.com/

FIRST AID GEAR AND TRAINING

The following organizations and retailers will help you obtain the training and gear necessary to be an effective first aid practitioner should a situation arise. Even if you don't have all the preferred training at this time, having a thorough first aid available during an emergency can allow another person with more advanced training to render immediate care. It's strongly encouraged to have a complete kit at home, in the car, and in your gear when outdoors.

RED CROSS
In addition to training in first aid and CPR, the Red Cross carries a full line of emergency kits and first aid supplies.
https://www.redcross.org/take-a-class
https://www.redcross.org/store/preparedness
https://www.redcross.org/store/first-aid-supplies

SKINNY MEDIC
Here is another great source of gear and information, as well as classes.
https://shop.skinnymedic.com/
http://www.skinnymedic.com/

CENTERS FOR DISEASE CONTROL AND PREVENTION

Here you will find the official government site covering a multitude of health-related topics. https://www.cdc.gov/

WILDERNESS MEDICAL ASSOCIATES

Here you will find courses and information from one of the most respected wilderness medicine schools in the country. If you are serious about learning the skills to deal with injuries in remote locations, these are the people to contact. https://www.wildmed.com/

COMMUNITY EMERGENCY RESPONSE TEAM (CERT)

Now found in all 50 states, C.E.R.T. teams help train volunteers in the fields of search and rescue, disaster medicine, emergency preparedness, and fire prevention. We are both part of our county's teams, and encourage anyone with an interest in this field to contact their county's emergency manager to see what opportunities are available. Classes are available for all skill and age groups. https://www.ready.gov/community-emergency-response-team

When it comes to keeping medical and first aid gear on hand in your house or other locations, we suggest utilizing the rewards card programs at retailers such as CVS, Rite Aid, Walgreens, or any other chain store in your region. Often times, they will send online coupons for up to 40% off one item or, in some cases, your total purchase. You can spend a little each week, and over the course of a few months, you will accumulate a good supply of medical gear. https://www.cvs.com/ • https://www.riteaid.com/ • https://www.walgreens.com/

While it's advisable to build your own first aid kit so that you can customize it to your specific needs, there are some reputable companies that produce quality, pre-assembled first aid kits. I own a few of the Adventure Medical kits, and have added some of my own gear to them to customize them to my needs. https://www.adventuremedicalkits.com/ • https://first-aid-product.com/first-aid-kits-cabinets.html • https://www.mfasco.com/first-aid-kits/

If you prefer organic salves to store-bought creams and gels, I heartily recommend Nicole's line of products, available online. I have some of her first aid and bug bite salve in the first aid kit that I keep in my vehicle. https://www.nicoleapelian.com/dr-nicoles-apothecary/

RECOMMENDED READING

Here are some books that Nicole and I recommend on preparedness, first aid, and the outdoors in general.

A Walk in the Woods
- by Bill Bryson

You may have seen the movie with Robert Redford and Nick Nolte, but the book is every bit as entertaining. If you've ever thought about striking out on a trip on the Appalachian Trail, this book is a humorous must read.

https://www.amazon.com/Walk-Woods-Rediscovering-America-Appalachian/dp/0307279464?crid=VPOJ2T1JY7OS&keywords=a+walk+in+the+woods+by+bill+bryson&qid=1539962096&s=Books&sprefix=a+walk+%2Cstripbooks%2C154&sr=1-1&ref=sr_1_1

Will You Be Ready? The Family Man's Guide to Basic Preparedness
- by Shawn Clay

Geared towards dads and husbands, I wrote this book to encourage men to make sure to plan contingencies for unexpected events that may dramatically impact their families. With the included checklists, having a plan and the right gear is easily accomplished.

https://www.amazon.com/Will-You-Be-Ready-Preparedness/dp/1537796631?keywords=shawn+clay&qid=1539962388&s=Sports+%26+Outdoors&sr=8-1&ref=sr_1_1

It's About More Than Just The Gear: Examining The Overlooked Aspects of Preparedness
- by Shawn Clay

In this book, I address the common phenomenon among the preparedness community of buying up all kinds of gear and gadgets, and then not pursuing the knowledge and skills necessary to successfully use them and teach others. As you will quickly see with this book, there is more to living a prepared lifestyle than just having a closet full of gear.

https://www.amazon.com/About-More-Than-Just-Gear/dp/1548002917?keyword s=shawn+clay&qid=1539962388&s=Sports+%26+Outdoors&sr=8-2&ref=sr_1_2

Audubon Society Field Guides

These field guides are available for nearly every animal and plant species imaginable. With full color photos and extensive information on habitat, behavior, etc., these guides set the gold standard for learning about all of the different outdoor life around you.

https://www.audubon.org/national-audubon-society-field-guides

There are literally thousands of books available on the topic of first aid. To help you whittle that list down, here is a helpful link to 22 highly recommended Emergency & Survival First Aid books:

https://morethanjustsurviving.com/best-first-aid-books/

National Geographic Guide to National Parks of the United States
By National Geographic

This helpful guide will allow you to plan and map out a trip to any one of our nation's wonderful national parks. A wonderful resource to help plan that family vacation of a lifetime.

https://www.amazon.com/National-Geographic-Guide-United-States/ dp/1426208693

National Geographic Guide to State Parks of the United States
By National Geographic

This companion guide to the National Park Guide details state parks available throughout the 50 states. Great for planning a day trip or weekend camping trip.

https://www.amazon.com/National-Geographic-Guide-United-States/dp/1426208898

Botany in a Day: The Patterns Method of Plant Identification: An Herbal Field Guide to Plant Families
By Thomas J. Elpel

http://www.hopspress.com/Books/Botany_in_a_Day.htm

Plants of the Pacific Northwest Coast
By Jim Pojar and Andy MacKinnon

https://www.amazon.com/Plants-Pacific-Northwest-Coast-Pojar/dp/1772130087

CHILDREN AND THE OUTDOORS

Here are some wonderful articles and websites, with links to additional resources, regarding the importance of children spending time in nature.

https://childmind.org/article/why-kids-need-to-spend-time-in-nature/

https://www.outdoorproject.com/blog-news/4-scientific-reasons-why-kids-should-be-outdoors

https://www.health.harvard.edu/blog/6-reasons-children-need-to-play-out-side-2018052213880

MAPS

Maps of your area can come in very handy when you are in a situation where GPS is spotty. I would recommend both road maps and topographic maps. Here are some links to help you obtain both types.

Rand McNally has been making road maps for over 100 years. I have one in each vehicle to serve as a backup if the GPS fails.

https://www.randmcnally.com/

The USGS (United States Geological Survey) has a variety of topographic maps available for purchase through their website. I would suggest picking one up of your area or the area you plan on spending time in.

https://store.usgs.gov/maps

LOCAL PRIVATE RESOURCES AND EDUCATION

Often times, you may have wonderful resources that are right in your hometown. Privately-funded nature reserves and educational centers can provide an oasis in the midst of the hustle and bustle of a major city where visitors can experience wildlife and open country. I am fortunate in the area where I live that I have access to Reflection Riding Arboretum and Nature Center and Audubon Acres. The Nature Center covers 317 acres at the foot of Lookout Mountain and includes 15 miles of trails where visitors can experience wildlife in their native habitat. There is also an educational center where visitors can learn more about the native wildlife of the region. In addition, they are one of only 42 centers worldwide that run a Red Wolf endangered species program. The staff here is knowledgeable and truly have the heart of a teacher.

Not far from the Nature Center is Audubon Acres, which houses the 130 acre Elise Chapin Wildlife Sanctuary. Here, visitors will find five miles of walking trails, picnic areas, and creeks to explore. These places are one of the many features that make the Chattanooga, TN region a wonderful place to live. I would encourage readers to check into their areas and see if there are similar facilities in their locales as well.

https://reflectionriding.org
https://www.chattanoogaaudubon.org/audubon-acres.html

Many cities and towns are now structuring development around nature, with a focus on preservation and environmental stewardship. Habitat destruction can threaten animal populations and responsible planning can help lessen the impact. Consider becoming active in any local land trust or preservation groups and ensure that natural areas are around to enjoy for generations to come. Here are a few of my local examples to check out:

LULA LAKE LAND TRUST
https://www.lulalake.org/

THE LAND TRUST FOR TENNESSEE
https://landtrusttn.org/

A quick online search of your area will likely turn up a similar non-profit group, so definitely take advantage of the resources that may be right at your backdoor!

SPECIAL THANKS

Shawn Clay - I would like to thank my family for supporting me in my writing. They know it's my passion and I could not ask for a better support system. I would also like to thank Nicole for undertaking this project with me. As a fan of both her and the series Alone, it's an honor to be able to work with her and count her as a friend. In a world where fake, scripted television shows masquerade as "reality", she is the real deal. I would also like to thank everyone who has read my books. Without you readers, this journey would never have progressed to where it is today. Finally, I would like to thank all of my friends, both old and new, who helped out with providing the photos for this book. There is a listing in the back with credits, but I just want to say a heartfelt thanks to everyone who provided pictures, as there were so many wonderful submissions that it was genuinely difficult to decide which ones to use. This kind of support is what keeps us small authors going, and I hope you all continue to follow me in all the books to come!

Nicole Apelian - I would like to thank my kids for their love, joy and their independent spirits. I deeply thank my co-author Shawn for both his friendship and his dedication to writing this book. I couldn't have asked for a better partner in this endeavor. I owe a huge gratitude to my step-father, who fueled my passion for the outdoors, and to my mom, who accepts who I am without question and who is always there for me. To all my mentors over the years - thank you! I have learned so much from you all and I hope I do you justice when I teach. A final huge thanks to Mother Nature and the deep connection I have with the outdoors. I hope that this book helps you to get outside with your families and enjoy all nature has to offer!

PHOTOGRAPHY AND COVER DESIGN

Nicole and I would like to thank the many people who contributed photographs for this book. Our only regret is that there was not enough room to use all of them, as there were so many wonderful submissions. Without your help, this project would not have been possible! Many thanks also to David Sparks of Hawthorne Media Group in Portland, Oregon for his cover design and book layout. You can view his work at www.hawthornemediagroup.com.

CHAPTER 2 - POISONOUS PLANTS

Poison Ivy #1 - Pixabay.com

Poison Ivy #2 - Nick Baker

Poison Ivy #3 - Forest Peace Tree-Hugger

Poison Ivy #4 - Sarah Spray

Poison Oak #1 - Lona Montgomery Gibbs

Poison Oak #2 - Lona Montgomery Gibbs

Poison Sumac #1 - Andy Jones

Poison Sumac #2 - Andy Jones

Stinging Nettle #1 - Nicole Apelian

Stinging Nettle #2 - Nicole Apelian

Dock - Thomas J. Elpel

Wood Nettle - Katy Chayka, www.MinnesotaWildflowers.info

Ragweed - Thomas J. Elpel

Giant Hogweed #1 - Adobe Stock Image

Giant Hogweed #2 - Pixabay.com

Giant Hogweed Rash - Photo taken by Bob Kleinberg and provided by NYSDEC

Wild Parsnip #1 - Adobe Stock Image

Wild Parsnip #2 - Robert Cornelius

CHAPTER 3 - INFURIATING INSECTS

Ants - University of Nebraska at Lincoln

Acrobat Ants - University of Nebraska at Lincoln

Carpenter Ants - University of Nebraska at Lincoln

Pavement Ants - University of Nebraska at Lincoln

Fire Ants - University of Nebraska at Lincoln

Honey Bee #1 - Matt Adderholt

Honey Bee #2 - Pixabay.com

African Bee #1 - Niculae Silviu Cristian

African Bee #2 - Pixabay.com

Bumble Bee #1 - Angie Marie's Photography

Bumble Bee #2 - Pixabay.com

Wasps - University of Nebraska at Lincoln

Bald-faced Hornet #1 - Adobe Stock Image

Bald-faced Hornet #2 - Pixabay.com
European Hornet #1 - Adobe Stock Image
European Hornet #2 - Pixabay.com
Paper Wasps - University of Nebraska at Lincoln
Yellowjackets - University of Nebraska at Lincoln
Mosquitos - University of Nebraska at Lincoln
Saddleback Caterpillar - University of Nebraska at Lincoln
Hag Moth Caterpillar - Brody Joe Thomassen
Puss Caterpillar - Brody Joe Thomassen
Stinging Rose Caterpillar - Niculae Silviu Cristian
Spiny Elm Caterpillar - Jack Bowling
White Flannel Caterpillar - Niculae Silviu Cristian
Crowned Slug Caterpillar - Brody Joe Thomassen
Io Moth Caterpillar - Brody Joe Thomassen
White-Marked Tussock Caterpillar - University of Nebraska at Lincoln
Buck Moth Caterpillar - Going On, Going On - Flickr user
Scorpion #1 - Niculae Silviu Cristian
Scorpion #2 - Rocky Hollow
Brown Recluse - University of Nebraska at Lincoln
Black Widow - University of Nebraska at Lincoln
Hobo Spider - University of Nebraska at Lincoln
Yellow Sac Spider - University of Nebraska at Lincoln
Deer Fly - University of Nebraska at Lincoln
Horse Fly - University of Nebraska at Lincoln
Stable Fly - University of Nebraska at Lincoln
Black Fly - University of Nebraska at Lincoln
Greenhead Fly - bitingflytrap.com
Biting Midge - University of Nebraska at Lincoln
American Dog Tick - University of Nebraska at Lincoln
Blacklegged Tick - University of Nebraska at Lincoln
Brown Dog Tick - University of Nebraska at Lincoln
Gulf Coast Tick - Steven Mickletz
Lone Star Tick - University of Nebraska at Lincoln
Rocky Mountain Wood Tick - University of Nebraska at Lincoln
Western Blacklegged Tick - Eric Engh

Centipede - University of Nebraska at Lincoln
Millipede - Pixabay.com
Leech - Niculae Silviu Cristian
Chigger - University of Nebraska at Lincoln
Chigger Bites - Mark Merriwether Vorderbruggen

CHAPTER 4 - CRITTERS THAT WALK AND SLITHER

Cougar #1 - Brenda Bean
Cougar #2 - Brenda Bean
Grizzly #1 - Brenda Bean
Grizzly #2 - Brenda Bean
Black Bear #1 - Nigel Dawson
Black Bear #2 - Nigel Dawson
Wolves #1 - William G. Moore
Wolves #2 - Brenda Bean
Wild Boar #1- Robert Dix
Wild Boar #2 - Ben Locke
Racoon #1 - Nick Baker
Racoon #2 - Pixabay.com
Skunk #1 - Niculae Silviu Cristian
Skunk #2 - Pixabay.com
Bat #1 - Niculae Silviu Cristian
Bat #2 - Pixabay.com
Coyote #1 - Nick Baker
Coyote #2 - Pixabay.com
Fox #1 - Angela Swiss
Fox #2 - Rick Pearson
Diamondback Rattlesnake #1 - Nick Baker
Diamondback Rattlesnake #2 - Nick Baker
Timber Rattlesnake #1 - Nick Baker
Timber Rattlesnake #2 - Nick Baker
Pygmy Rattlesnake #1 - John Howell
Pygmy Rattlesnake #2 - snakeremovaltrap.com
Prairie Rattlesnake #1 - Adobe Stock Image
Prairie Rattlesnake #2 - Pixabay.com
Sidewinder Rattlesnake #1 - Niculae Silviu Cristian

Sidewinder Rattlesnake #2 - Pixabay.com

Timber Rattlesnake - Shawn Clay

Copperhead #1 - Nick Baker

Copperhead #2 - Nick Baker

Cottonmouth #1 - Nick Baker

Cottonmouth #2 - Nick Baker

Northern Water Snake - Shawn Clay

Coral Snake #1 - Ian Deery

Coral Snake #2 - Ian Deery

American Alligator #1 - "Achim Raschka / CC-BY-SA-4.0" //commons.wikimedia.org/wiki/File:A_miss._berlin_3.JPG)

CHAPTER 5 - WICKED WEATHER

Frostbite #1 - Niculae Silviu Cristian

Frostbite #2 - Niculae Silviu Cristian

Sunburn #1 - Niculae Silviu Cristian

Sunburn #2 - Adam Jacobson

Wildfire #1 - Pixabay.com

Wildfire #2 - Pixabay.com

Lightning #1 - Niculae Silviu Cristian

Lightning #2 - Angela Swiss

APPENDIX

SIX COMMON MEDICINAL PLANTS & LICHENS FOR USE IN THE FIELD

Mullein #1 - Thomas J. Elpel

Mullein #2 - Thomas J. Elpel

Plantain #1 - Thomas J. Elpel

Plantain #2 - F.D. Richards

Stinging Nettle - Kruscha - Pixabay.com

Usnea #1 - Jason Hollinger

Usnea #2 - Bernd Haynold

Willow #1 - Public Domain - Wikimedia

Willow #2 - Evelyn Simak

Yarrow #1 - Thomas J. Elpel

Yarrow #2 - Open Clipart Vectors - Pixabay.com

NOTES

NOTES

_____

_____

_____

_____

_____

_____

_____

_____

_____

_____

_____

_____

_____

_____

_____

_____

_____

_____

_____

_____

_____

_____

_____

_____

_____

_____

_____

_____

_____

_____

_____

_____

_____

NOTES

NOTES

NOTES

NOTES

NOTES

NOTES

NOTES

NOTES

BASIC EMERGENCY FIELD KIT CHECKLIST
AS RECOMMENDED BY NICOLE APELIAN

FIRE
- [ ] Ferro rod
- [ ] Lighter
- [ ] Fire starting tinder
- [ ] Fresnel lens

SIGNALING
- [ ] Map compass
- [ ] Emergency whistle
- [ ] Signal mirror
- [ ] Bright neon flag / clothing
- [ ] Small flashlight with extra batteries

WATER
- [ ] Steel water bottle kit with nesting cup for cooking
- [ ] Water bags
- [ ] Water purification tablets
- [ ] Sawyer Mini water filter

SHELTER
- [ ] Paracord - at least 20'
- [ ] Wire saw
- [ ] Emergency rain poncho
- [ ] Emergency tarp / shelter sheet
- [ ] Mylar blanket

FOOD PROCUREMENT
- [ ] 28 gauge brass snare wire
- [ ] Fishing line and hooks

OTHER
- [ ] Mora Knife (or other type)
- [ ] Extra small knife / saw combo
- [ ] Small sewing kit
- [ ] Local area map

FIRST AID / MEDICAL
- [ ] Emergency medication (anti-diarrheal, aspirin, Ibuprofen, Benadryl, prescription medication)
- [ ] 3 Bandaids (minimum)
- [ ] 2 Butterfly closures (minimum)
- [ ] First aid salve
- [ ] RevMedX and/or SWAT-T tourniquet
- [ ] Chito-Sam and/or Israeli Bandage

"I believe that there is a subtle magnetism in Nature, which, if we
unconsciously yield to it, will direct us aright."
– Henry David Thoreau

"In the presence of nature, a wild delight runs
through the man, in spite of real sorrows."
– Ralph Waldo Emerson

"Nature gives to every time and season
some beauties of its own."
– Charles Dickens

"I go to Nature to be soothed and healed,
and to have my senses put together."
– John Burroughs

"There is a way that nature speaks, that land speaks.
Most of the time we are simply not patient enough,
quiet enough, to pay attention to the story."
– Linda Hogan

"Earth and sky, woods and fields, lakes and rivers, the
mountain and the sea, are excellent schoolmasters, and teach
of us more than we can ever learn from books."
– John Lubbock

"Look deep into nature, and then you will
understand everything better."
– Albert Einstein

CPSIA information can be obtained
at www.ICGtesting.com
Printed in the USA
LVHW052342220620
658659LV00006B/487

9 780578 489988